# making the

# CUT

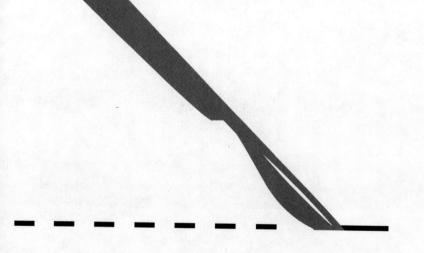

# *making the*
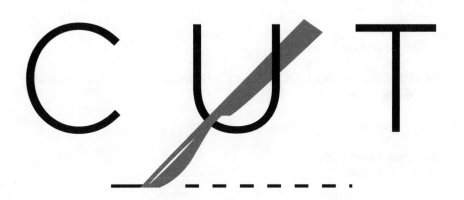

# CUT

Ten Things You Should Consider

## Before Having Plastic Surgery

# DARSHAN SHAH, MD

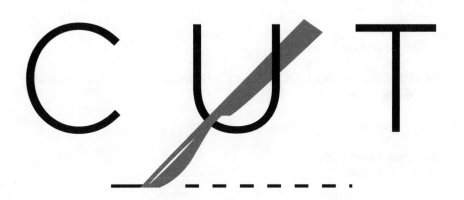

Published by Advantage, Charleston, South Carolina.
Member of Advantage Media Group.

ADVANTAGE is a registered trademark and the Advantage colophon is a trademark of Advantage Media Group, Inc.

Printed in the United States of America.

ISBN: 978-1-59932-494-4
LCCN: 2016942000

Book design by George Stevens.

This publication is designed to provide accurate and authoritative information in regard to the subject matter covered. It is sold with the understanding that the publisher is not engaged in rendering legal, accounting, or other professional services. If legal advice or other expert assistance is required, the services of a competent professional person should be sought.

All opinions in this book are for you to discuss with your own physician. None of the authors of this book is your physician and therefore cannot give you medical advice. This book is to serve as points of discussion between you and your doctor, and should not be taken as medical advice.

Advantage Media Group is proud to be a part of the Tree Neutral® program. Tree Neutral offsets the number of trees consumed in the production and printing of this book by taking proactive steps such as planting trees in direct proportion to the number of trees used to print books. To learn more about Tree Neutral, please visit **www.treeneutral.com.** To learn more about Advantage's commitment to being a responsible steward of the environment, please visit **www.advantagefamily.com/green**

Advantage Media Group is a publisher of business, self-improvement, and professional development books and online learning. We help entrepreneurs, business leaders, and professionals share their Stories, Passion, and Knowledge to help others Learn & Grow. Do you have a manuscript or book idea that you would like us to consider for publishing? Please visit **advantagefamily.com** or call **1.866.775.1696.**

*A special thanks to my family and all of my patients.*

# Contents

# PART 2

## What You Should Know before Going Forward

# Introduction

The field of plastic surgery has undergone a major transformation in the past few decades. When plastic surgery was first gaining popularity in the 1970s, it was primarily the domain of movie stars, models, and the elite. By the late 1980s, more and more people chose to have plastic surgery, as they saw their favorite celebrity have a successful outcome. Still, the appeal was limited because plastic surgery was so expensive and required a significant amount of time and money.

By the turn of the twenty-first century, a revolution in plastic surgery was underway. Stories about the growing number of procedures and their amazing results flooded the various media outlets; popular primetime television shows, such as *Extreme Makeover, Dr. 90210*, and others, helped make plastic surgery a hot topic around dinner tables and hair salons across America. With plastic surgery on everyone's minds as a viable alternative for the "regular person," it was finally becoming more accessible to a larger group of consumers as costs became more reasonable and the recovery process shortened due to advances in surgical techniques. As the demand for plastic surgery rapidly increased, more doctors started doing it. An increase in the supply of well-trained plastic surgeons also helped bring prices down to levels that a larger number of Americans could afford.

At about the same time, geographic availability began expanding. Whereas plastic surgery had originally been concentrated in certain areas—mainly New York City and Beverly Hills—doctors began offering these surgical procedures to patients in cities across America. This convergence of media exposure, accessibility in terms of cost, and geographic availability led to a huge expansion of the industry that continues today. Every year the number of cosmetic procedures expands, and plastic surgery has also become a global phenomenon, with hot spots in South Korea, China, the Middle East, and South America.

As the number of people opting for plastic surgery grew, general perceptions about it changed, as well. Plastic surgery was no longer something reserved for Hollywood celebrities, fashion models, and the very wealthy, all of whom were considered "vain" by the majority of the population. Now, plastic surgery is viewed as something that practically anyone can do.

For example, today we see many women choosing the "mommy makeover": American mothers who have finished having children just want to get their prepregnancy body back. While that notion was once considered vain, many women today feel that it's practically a rite of passage. After all, why should they live with stretch marks and deflated breasts if they don't have to?

Another rising trend is happening in the workplace. Because people are working later and later in their lives, many feel that in order to remain competitive, especially in sales or other highly visible positions, they need to look as young as they feel. With the advent of minimally invasive procedures to eliminate wrinkles from the face, having cosmetic work done is considered by some to be "maintenance," something they do on a regular basis to maintain their viability in the workforce as they age, not unlike coloring hair or getting teeth whitened.

The days of plastic surgery only being a realistic option for the rich and famous are over; now virtually anyone has the opportunity of a cosmetic enhancement if they so choose.

It is clear that the revolution in plastic surgery that began at the turn of the century has resulted in a snowball effect in terms of improving attitudes toward it among Americans. As plastic and cosmetic procedures became more easily accessible, a shift in perception about these procedures soon followed. In 2011 the American Society for Aesthetic Plastic Surgery conducted a survey that found that more than half of Americans (51 percent) had no problem with the idea of cosmetic surgery, and 67 percent said they would *not be* embarrassed if their friends and family knew they had had cosmetic surgery.

The growing number of Americans undergoing plastic surgery procedures indicates that those considering it likely have a friend, neighbor, colleague, or family member who has had one done. Word of mouth is the biggest reason why the numbers continue to climb year after year, both in terms of how many people are having it done and how many people approve of the idea. Talking to people who

---

**Who's Having Plastic Surgery in America?**

The number of people having cosmetic procedures rose in 2015 from the previous year in every single age group, from teens (aged thirteen to nineteen years old) to people over fifty-five. The numbers also rose among both men and women and among every ethnic group.

- 12.7 million cosmetic procedures were performed in the USA in 2015—up from 10.5 million the previous year

- $13.5 billion was spent on cosmetic procedures, up 5.5 percent from the previous year

- 6 percent rise in the number of procedures among people over forty

- 5 percent rise in the number of procedures performed on men

*Statistics from the American Society for Aesthetic Plastic Surgery: *2015 Plastic Surgery Statistics Report*

have had plastic surgery reveals just how easy it is to get procedures done. Hearing about great results, quick and easy recovery times, and the renewed senses of self-confidence and self-esteem that follow a procedure make having plastic surgery feel like a viable possibility.

Alongside all of this has been a steady stream of technological advancements that makes plastic surgery less risky and less costly than ever before. One of the first minimally invasive procedures was Botox®, which was approved by the FDA in 2002 for the treatment of frown lines. That revolutionized the industry by convincing even more people that they too could improve their appearance with a quick office visit and no downtime. After Botox® came many other types of procedures such as dermal fillers and laser procedures that capitalized on the idea of the quick fix. This spawned a whole new industry of minimally invasive cosmetic procedures, as well as the medical spa.

Currently, there's a huge push in research and development in the field of cosmetic procedures, in large part due to the fact that it's mostly a cash business. Innovation occurs at a rapid rate because the field is not bogged down by insurance and government regulations in the same way most other fields of medicine are. That means there are new advancements happening all the time.

With so much happening so rapidly in our field, confusion and doubt understandably set in. There is so much information out there, how do you choose what is best? The question also arises, "How do I avoid a botched surgery, devastating complication, or less-than-optimal results?" This book attempts to answer that question in a comprehensive, easy-to-understand manner.

Not only is choosing the right doctor and right procedure an important decision but patients must first take a step back and truly examine why they are considering plastic surgery in the first place. Are they in the right state of mind? Is this the right time in their lives?

Do they have the right support? Despite the television portrayals of plastic surgery being a quick fix that can change someone's life within a thirty-minute infomercial, the truth is that having surgery is a big deal, and you should treat it as such.

## About Me and My Practice

When I first graduated from medical school, I decided to train in general surgery. I learned and performed a number of serious, life-saving procedures like major trauma surgery, abdominal and chest operations, the removal of cancers, and other major procedures. After five years of this incredible experience, I decided I wanted to take on a new challenge. I saw plastic surgery as the most difficult learning opportunity that surgery could offer because it was an emerging field at the time. The depth of knowledge of human anatomy and the extreme amounts of manual dexterity and skill required for the operations provided me with the inspiration to spend another two years at the Mayo Clinic learning this skill. I was intrigued by the fact that people could assess the results of their surgery just by looking at themselves in the mirror. Whether or not I had been successful was right out there for everyone to see and judge. I considered that the ultimate test, so I decided to specialize in plastic surgery.

I then trained at the Mayo Clinic in Rochester, Minnesota, which is considered one of the top hospitals in the country. I wanted to learn from the best, so I spent two years doing a fellowship in plastic surgery where I saw all sorts of revolutionary procedures, both cosmetic and reconstructive. After I finished my training, I started my own practice, which took off rather quickly. From there, I partnered with more physicians and opened more offices. One of the primary reasons our physician practice, Beautologie Cosmetic Surgery & Laser Center, grew so rapidly was because we adopted a customer service mind-set. We veered away from the traditional doctor's office environment, where patients have long wait times and limited communication with their doctor. We made it our mission to really focus on the customer service aspect of serving our patients and making it a beautiful, amazing experience that is life changing in its own right. Today we operate four offices in California, and we have plans to expand in the near future.

My colleagues at Beautologie and I were attracted to the field of plastic surgery because it's different from all of the other medical fields out there. It's about more than just becoming a skilled surgeon, though that's important too. Beyond that, we have the privilege of really diving into our patients' lives—of learning about their dreams and ambitions and about their levels of self-confidence. With plastic surgery, it's important for surgeons to not only be technically skilled but also to be skilled communicators. We believe it is extremely important for our surgeons to fully understand the patients' expectations—specifically, what kind of a change they're expecting, not only physically but also in their lives and relationships. These are the kinds of things that we talk about every single day in our practice with almost every one of our patients.

So every plastic surgery procedure we perform starts with a conversation. It often results in a deep conversation that brings out a lot of fears and life issues concerning self-confidence, relationships, feelings of self-worth, and even childhood issues that often began with teasing about a physical aspect of their body or face. Many of these issues are difficult for people to talk about, but we understand how important it is to bring these feelings out into the open in order to have a productive discussion about the surgery. It also gives us an opportunity to inject realism into the conversation, to establish realistic expectations of what the procedure can physically achieve for our patients and also what type of changes they can expect in their life as a result. For example, plastic surgery won't bring back your estranged lover, but it might give you renewed self-confidence to move on to the next phase of your life.

That's why this book is set up the way it is. Right up front I wanted to address the ten biggest reasons *not* to have plastic surgery so people can really think about what their motivations are before they proceed. I think it's much more beneficial to present the reasons to not do it first and then, if all those reasons are addressed, to understand how to move forward in order to get great results, both physically and psychologically. When someone opts for plastic surgery for all the right reasons and is realistic about the results, that person is set up for success. Over the years, I've seen thousands of patients who have really undergone a profound life change in terms of how they feel about themselves and how they see themselves as a result of having a successful procedure. I'm privileged to have shared in that journey thousands of times. It is my passion to educate and connect with my patients, and I hope this book conveys that passion.

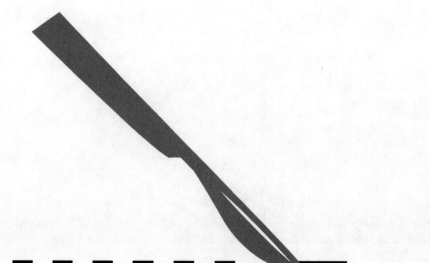

# PART 1

----------

## Reasons That You May Not Be a Good Candidate for Plastic Surgery

H aving plastic surgery means not only making a permanent change in your appearance but also in your life. You will be surprised at the exponential changes you will feel in your self-esteem, relationships, daily activities—in virtually every aspect of your life! That's why I believe it's critically important people really understand why they want to undergo plastic surgery. Sometimes, when performed for the wrong reasons, it's a setup for an unhappy result.

In this section, I outline ten of the most common *wrong* reasons why people choose to have plastic surgery. If you go through these ten reasons and address each one of them honestly, you will have taken a huge step in setting yourself up for a great result and a positive life change. To really make sure you *get it*, I have included a short quiz at the end of each chapter to help you determine if you have done enough to address each particular issue. If you pass the quiz, you will know you're ready to move on to the next chapter. And if you pass all ten, you will know that you have considered pretty much everything in your power to set yourself up for a great experience!

# Not Healthy

T he number-one reason *not* to have plastic surgery is ill health. This is an absolutely essential consideration. If you are not healthy and you undergo any kind of elective surgery, not just plastic surgery, you are setting yourself up for potential complications, including not making it through the procedure. Of course, no one wants to undergo an elective procedure only to end up dying or being hospitalized for a long period of time. You want to have a successful surgery and a normal recovery so that you may enjoy the results afterward! Ensuring that you're healthy enough for surgery is absolutely essential and the number-one concern that you should have. Remember that virtually all cosmetic plastic surgery is "elective." That means it is completely *your* choice to undergo the procedure, and we have total control of the timing of the procedure. It is a huge mistake to undergo an elective procedure *when* your physical condition is not optimized for success.

In order to make sure you're healthy enough for elective surgery, you should first go to your regular doctor for a medical checkup. If your doctor doesn't perform the type of pre-surgery clearance exams that will prepare you for plastic surgery, you should find a doctor who does.

In this era of personal empowerment, you must, as the patient, take charge of your own health. Don't rely on the doctor to make all the right decisions for you. Sometimes, the doctor may forget to ask you about your health history, check blood work, and so on. It is your right to ask questions, so ask, "How do you know that I am healthy enough to undergo surgery?"

It's also very important that the primary care doctor doing your evaluation is comfortable with your decision to have plastic surgery. Many times, physicians bring their own values and attitudes to the discussion. They might say, right off the bat, "Oh, you don't need a procedure like that," or "Don't do something like that." You don't want a doctor who is negative about your plan to have plastic surgery. It's your decision. If your doctor is negative about it, for personal reasons, you might consider finding a different doctor to complete your medical evaluation. Of course, if it's not safe for you to undergo a procedure at the time, your doctor should tell you that, and you should definitely listen. But again, if your doctor takes the attitude that you don't need the procedure and he thinks you look fine the way you are, *and you disagree*, then you're starting off on the wrong foot.

Once you find a general practitioner or family practice doctor with whom you're comfortable talking about this subject, there are certain health factors you want to be sure he/she evaluates. In our practice we have a formal letter that we have all of our patients give to their doctors to make sure they do the appropriate presurgical checks. It is important to understand that most plastic surgery procedures are done under general anesthesia, which can put stress on your body, especially if you have other concurrent health issues. Therefore, you should confirm that you're considered low risk before you undergo any procedure.

Following is a list of evaluation criteria that your doctor should assess to determine whether you are in good enough health to have a procedure. This doesn't mean that you have to be in "perfect health." If you scan the following checklist, you may wonder what it means for you if you have diabetes, for example, or asthma. The answer is that having one of these conditions doesn't mean you *can't* have an elective procedure. What it does mean is that your health condition must be under control (i.e. "optimized") and both your primary physician and your plastic surgeon are well aware of it prior to surgery.

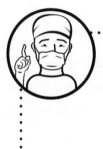

**Dr. Shah Recommends**

Get your "good health" medical clearance before you see the plastic surgeon.

### Medical Evaluation Checklist

- *Cardiac evaluation*: A cardiac evaluation should be done and, if indicated, an EKG test. This tells the doctor if your heart is healthy enough for you to undergo surgery. This is a major risk factor when undergoing surgery because some of the medication given to you for anesthesia can have various effects on your heart. If your heart is not strong enough, or has other issues such as arrhythmias, you could have a problem with anesthesia. If you have a history of heart attacks, high blood pressure, any kind of chest pain with exertion, or an abnormal heartbeat, you need to bring it up with your doctor prior to surgery.

- *Vascular evaluation:* A vascular evaluation is one way of checking to make sure you are not at risk of having a stroke during surgery. If you have had any of the symptoms of TIA (transient ischemic attack) or stroke, then this should be brought up with your doctor prior to surgery.

- *Pulmonary evaluation:* This is to make sure that your lungs are in good working order. Most doctors will listen to your lungs and make sure you don't have any pulmonary issues such as asthma COPD. If you do, your doctor may have you get a chest X-ray prior to surgery. You should also stop smoking and avoid nicotine for a period before and after a surgical procedure. (You'll find much more on this subject under Reason #3.)

- *Diabetes evaluation:* Diabetes is a huge problem for postoperative healing. If you have a problem with diabetes, your healing will be slow or problematic. That doesn't mean you can't have surgeries, but you must have your diabetic care optimized beforehand. One way a doctor knows that your diabetic care is optimized and that your blood sugar is under reasonable control is by performing a blood test called the HgA1c. In our practice, we like to see the HgA1c level under seven to feel reasonably safe that you will have good healing after surgery. If there's any indication that your blood sugar is not under good control, you should get it under good control prior to surgery.

- *Deep venous thrombosis or pulmonary embolism risk evaluation:* This is about assessing your risk for getting a blood clot in your legs. If you've ever had a blood clot in your leg, if you're taking birth control pills, or if you have any other risk factors for having a deep venous thrombosis, you need to have that evaluated. For example, women who are in their forties, are overweight, and don't do any physical activity are at higher risk. Depending on what procedure they're having, women on birth control may be asked to pause them and use alternate methods of birth control prior to surgery to lower the risk.

- *Post-weight-loss patients:* Many patients have lost a lot of weight prior to plastic surgery, either through surgical means such as bariatric surgery or on their own. Sometimes, especially after bariatric surgery, patients have severe electrolyte, hydration, and anemia issues. Those all need to be addressed and treated before we do a procedure.

- *Blood work:* Blood work is important for everyone to have done before a surgical procedure because it can bring to light a number of health issues such as bleeding problems, anemia, and electrolyte problems, all of which could impede your surgery or your recovery. For example, one of the major contraindications to elective surgery is low hemoglobin (the molecule that carries oxygen to your tissues). In our practice, we recommend that your hemoglobin level be over twelve before undergoing any major elective surgery.

## Increasing Your Chance of a Positive Outcome

Being in good health is not just about making it through anesthesia successfully. It also has an impact on how well you recover and how nicely your incisions heal. One of the important things to realize about plastic surgery is that, sometimes, we remove a large amount of skin or lift a large amount of skin and put it back into place. If the blood supply to your skin is not optimized, you can get what we call "wound breakdown," an opening of your incisions, following surgery, which often leads to an infection. People with diabetes and other vascular issues, for example, are at high risk for infection and poor healing.

Sometimes, when you have an open wound, it has to heal secondarily, which means you protect it with wet gauze and then just let it heal on its own over the course of weeks. But that kind of healing may end up turning into an unsightly scar, which is disconcerting to most patients. Being medically optimized before surgery is extremely important for helping to prevent wound breakdown and your scarring from getting out of control. No one who undergoes plastic surgery is looking to end up with a bad scar, and neither is your surgeon! That's why, after the initial stages of healing, it's important to have the time and intention to take care of yourself and your incision so you maintain a good result. (We'll talk more about this consideration under Reason #8.)

## When Plastic Surgery Just Isn't a Good Idea

It's important to understand that if you are healthy, there is minimal risk in undergoing plastic surgery. You're not likely to have any type of problem either during or after your procedure. But there are some health problems that make undergoing plastic surgery absolutely contraindicated (should not be done). One of those conditions is a family history of something called "malignant hyperthermia," which is a life-threatening genetic disease where your body temperature goes out of control when you undergo anesthesia with some commonly used medications. If someone in your family has it, you need to be tested for it, and you really should stay away from having any type of unnecessary surgery, including plastic surgery.

In the medical profession, there's a criteria system that is used in almost every operating room called the American Society of Anesthesiologists criteria. If you've had serious health issues and you have a physical status classification of three or higher based on the ASA criteria, then you really should not be having elective surgery at this time. In fact, you really shouldn't be having surgery at all unless it's a medical emergency.

## The Critical Importance of a Preoperative Medical Evaluation

In 2007 it was big news when Donda West, mother to rapper Kanye West, died the day after undergoing plastic surgery. It's possible that this tragic outcome could have been avoided if she had gotten a proper medical clearance prior to surgery. No one checked her out medically beforehand, so her plastic surgeon didn't know about some of her medical issues, including preexisting coronary artery disease. She underwent an eight-hour surgery, after which she went home. Her pre-existing medical conditions, combined with a long surgical procedure, lead to her eventual demise. In our practice, we recommend that if you're going to have more than four hours of surgery, you should spend the night after it in the hospital under nursing supervision. Sadly, Ms. West is an example of someone who didn't set herself up to have a good result. It is unfortunate that her surgeon did not insist on a medical exam before surgery, which may have saved her life.

**ASA Physical Status 1** - A normal healthy patient

**ASA Physical Status 2** - A patient with mild systemic disease

**ASA Physical Status 3** - A patient with severe systemic disease

**ASA Physical Status 4** - A patient with severe systemic disease that is a constant threat to life

**ASA Physical Status 5** - A moribund patient who is not expected to survive without the operation

**ASA Physical Status 6** - A declared brain-dead patient whose organs are being removed for donor purposes

### Dr. Shah Recommends

Ask your doctor if it would be helpful for you to spend the night in a hospital or recovery center after surgery.

## Preoperative Medical Clearance

Following, as an example, is a copy of a letter we have patients give to their primary-care physicians to obtain the right medical clearance for plastic surgery. You can use it as a guideline to discuss with your own doctor to help ensure you're in good health prior to surgery.

Dear Doctor:

Your patient has made the voluntary decision to undergo a surgical procedure. In order to ensure patient safety, we would like to obtain your surgical clearance before we proceed with the surgery. The patient will be receiving general anesthesia for an outpatient procedure that will last approximately one to five hours. Most plastic surgery procedures are considered low to moderate risk.

Specifically, we would like the patient to be evaluated for at least the following items. Any other evaluations that would affect the patient, per your complete history and physical, which you deem necessary, are at your discretion. Thank you for your assistance in our goal of providing excellent patient care in the safest possible environment.

1. *Cardiac evaluation:* We would require at least an EKG. If you feel the patient's EKG or cardiac risk factors warrant a stress test, echo, angiogram, or other test, please obtain as well. Electrolyte levels, especially if the patient is on any medications, would be excellent. Hypertension must be under good control to proceed.

2. *Vascular evaluation:* If you feel that the patient is at risk for a CVA or other vascular complication, a carotid Doppler or other examination should be obtained.

3. *Pulmonary evaluation:* If there is any indication to obtain a chest X-ray, ABG, or PFT, please do so. All patients should be encouraged to stop smoking and avoid all forms of nicotine before their procedure.

4. *Diabetes evaluation:* Since diabetes can cause healing difficulties, we would like the patient to be under good control when about to undergo

a procedure. The HgAlc test results should be under seven within six months from the date of surgery. In addition, medication alteration may be necessary per your guidelines to prevent perioperative hypoglycemia.

5. *DVT/PE prophylaxis:* All patients who are to undergo a major liposuction or abdominoplasty will receive 40 mg of Lovenox prior to the procedure. Any other suggestions you have, based on the individual patient's risk factors, would be appreciated.

6. *Preoperative anemia:* We have noticed that many patients are anemic prior to surgery. An Hg/Hct and PT/PTT would be helpful during your examination to evaluate and correct any deficiencies well in advance of any surgical procedure.

7. *Post-gastric bypass patients:* As you know, these patients occasionally have severe electrolyte, hydration, and anemia issues. Please complete a comprehensive metabolic profile and CBC to evaluate and begin to treat vitamin and iron deficiencies as indicated.

8. *Other:* _____

_____

Of course, the preoperative clearance should not be limited to only the above evaluations. If you feel that there are other issues that preclude surgery, or should be brought to our attention, please do not hesitate to contact us. We truly appreciate your assistance in this matter. *After your evaluation, if you could have your office fax us copies of the EKG, lab work, history and physical, and a note from you, stating you feel it is okay to go ahead with the procedure, we would appreciate that.*

Sincerely,

------------------------------------------

### Dr. Shah Recommends

Don't rely too much on age to assess your overall health. That means that you shouldn't assume that because you're under forty, you're healthy enough for plastic surgery, or that because you're older, that you're not. Age is relative and plenty of people up to the age of sixty-five have plastic surgery all the time. The rule at our practice is that if you're over the age of sixty-five, we'll do your surgery in the hospital where we can observe you overnight afterward.

## Test Yourself

Make sure you can answer <u>yes</u> to all of these questions before you proceed with scheduling your plastic surgery procedure.

1. Have you had a medical evaluation done by your primary care physician within the last six months?

2. Did your medical evaluation cover all the points listed in the previous checklist?

3. Have you divulged to both your primary-care physician and your plastic surgeon all medical issues and surgical procedures you are having now and/or have had in the past?

4. Have you given a list of all your current and past medications (including supplements, herbal medications, etc.) to your primary-care physician and to your plastic surgeon?

5. Have you given a list of all of your medications and food and environmental allergies to your primary-care physician and your plastic surgeon?

6. Are you and your doctor confident that any medical issues you have are under control and that, overall, you are in good health for the procedure?

7. Did you ask, "What is my ASA physical status classification?" Is it two or under?

8. Did your surgeon discuss the risks of surgery with you?

9. Do you have health insurance to cover you in case you do have to go to the hospital for any reason after the surgery?

10. Does the person performing your anesthesia know your full medical history and have all the records of your medical clearance exam?

If you answered yes to all of these questions, you have passed this test. Congratulations! You are one step closer to getting your procedure!

— — — — — — — — — — — — — — —

# Obesity

O besity is often viewed as a reason to have plastic surgery, but that's a misconception. Plastic surgery cannot make an obese person skinny. What plastic surgery can do is remove problem areas of fat that you have trouble getting rid of with diet and exercise. It can also remove loose skin that occurs with aging, after losing weight, or after childbirth. But it's unrealistic to think that plastic surgery can make someone who's very overweight look thin.

That does not mean that if you are a little overweight, you can't look amazing with the help of plastic surgery. You absolutely can, but there's a threshold. We use the body mass index (BMI) as a guide when considering if someone is a good candidate for surgery. BMI is a guide based on your height and weight that helps us categorize your level of obesity.

## BMI Guidelines

In general, if your BMI is in the normal or slightly overweight range, it's okay to have plastic surgery. If your BMI is over thirty, which is the obese category, in most cases we recommend you lose weight and get your BMI to normal or close before you have a plastic surgery procedure. If your BMI is thirty-five to forty, you should probably not be having plastic surgery unless you've already had bariatric surgery for weight loss and you've lost as much weight as you can. If your BMI is over forty, plastic surgery is almost always contraindicated, and you need to pursue weight-loss options on your own before you undergo any type of plastic surgery procedure. You can consult the chart on this page to find out what your own BMI score is. The BMI chart is easy to use; just find your height on one axis, your weight on the other, and you have a number.

Why is your weight so important? The main reason we look at your BMI is that being obese directly affects your healing process after surgery. A number of large research studies have shown that people who are obese have a higher rate of wound breakdown complications in almost all surgical procedures than people who are not overweight. They are also at greater risk for complications such as blood clots, pneumonia, and seroma (a fluid collection that can develop under the skin). Basically, the risk of almost any complication after surgery increases if you're obese. People who are obese also experience longer recovery times, longer surgical times, and more postoperative infections.

One of the main problems with being overweight or obese before plastic surgery is that there is a much higher chance that you won't be happy with the results. There is only so much fat and skin that can be removed in surgery. Obesity hides fat under your muscles and around your organs (called "visceral fat") where we cannot physically remove it. This leads to less-than-optimal results and dissatisfaction in the end. Many people regret spending a great deal of money and time on the procedure only to have less-than-optimal results due to being overweight. They come to realize that it would have been much better to lose the weight before surgery.

## Know Your BMI

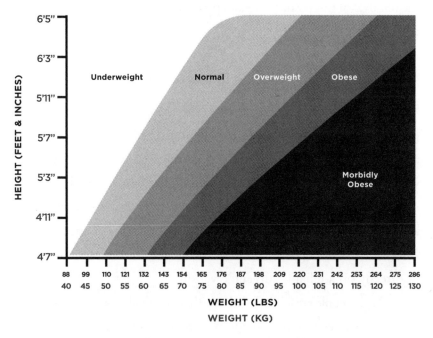

**HEIGHT (FEET & INCHES)**

6'5"
6'3"
5'11"
5'7"
5'3"
4'11"
4'7"

Underweight   Normal   Overweight   Obese

Morbidly Obese

| 88 | 99 | 110 | 121 | 132 | 143 | 154 | 165 | 176 | 187 | 198 | 209 | 220 | 231 | 242 | 253 | 264 | 275 | 286 |
| 40 | 45 | 50 | 55 | 60 | 65 | 70 | 75 | 80 | 85 | 90 | 95 | 100 | 105 | 110 | 115 | 120 | 125 | 130 |

**WEIGHT (LBS)**

**WEIGHT (KG)**

## Exceptions to the BMI Guidelines

There are some exceptions to these guidelines, specific situations in which an obese person *can* have plastic surgery. Someone with a BMI over thirty can, sometimes, have surgery to get tissue out of the way, such as a breast reduction. We don't necessarily have to wait for the weight loss before performing that kind of surgery, because, for some people, most of their extra weight is concentrated in their breasts. In these cases, a breast reduction really helps patients get down to a more comfortable size, which allows them to exercise more effectively.

Another exception involves panniculectomy: removal of a large fold of extra skin from underneath the abdomen where rashes can occur. Again, we perform that surgery to get the tissue out of the way so patients can be more mobile. Plastic surgeons will, sometimes, perform procedures under this circumstance, but they are considered more reconstructive than aesthetic because patients have it done mainly to get tissue out of the way so they can have a more productive life. In many cases, the removal of this tissue motivates patients to exercise and improve their dietary habits afterward, leading to more weight loss.

## Realistic Expectations

Something I do for all our patients who are considering any kind of plastic surgery is show them before and after photos of what can be achieved so they have realistic expectations of what's possible and what's not. I try to find a similar-looking patient in our large bank of before and after pictures so that the patient can see what can be achieved. When you are looking at before and after pictures on the Internet, it is imperative you look for images from a credible source or directly on a reliable surgeon's website.

Many people mistakenly believe that they will lose a lot of weight with these surgeries, but with liposuction or a tummy tuck, you'll rarely see a significant change on your bathroom scale. In fact, most people will actually weigh more immediately after surgery because of the swelling that occurs. (Of course, that extra weight will go away once the swelling goes down.) A typical specimen of the tissue we remove during these procedures only weighs two to five pounds. You might look as if you've lost twenty pounds because of the way the surgeon has contoured your body, but fat and skin don't weigh a lot per inch removed. For the most part, you can expect to lose less than five pounds on the scale even though you might look significantly different. That's why it's important that you're in an acceptable BMI range before the surgery, because having surgery alone is not going to do the trick.

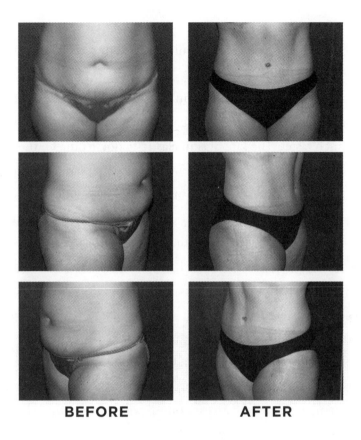

**BEFORE**       **AFTER**

## Weight-Loss Surgery

There are surgeries that can help with excess weight, but they are not usually done by plastic surgeons. If your goal is to lose a significant amount of weight on the scale, you should speak with a reputable doctor and consider weight-loss surgery (also called bariatric surgery) before plastic surgery, though it's important to understand that the two types of surgery often go hand-in-hand.

If your BMI is over forty and you really feel that there's no way you're going to lose the weight on your own, then it can be an option to pursue bariatric surgery. Bariatric surgery has become safer in recent years, and many people have had huge success with it. But beware: it's important to realize that while bariatric surgery can help you lose the weight, it may also cause a lot of loose skin, not just in your abdomen and your breasts but also in your face, your legs, your neck, your back, and so on.

Loose skin can also develop in people who lose weight on their own, but the effect is greater with bariatric surgery because the weight is lost much faster. The rate of skin elasticity doesn't match the rate of the weight loss, so you have more loose skin afterward compared to losing the weight on your own. Some people who undergo bariatric surgery are shocked at the amount of loose skin they have afterward. Some hate the loose skin more than they hated being overweight. On occasion, people say, "Gosh, I wish I never had the weight-loss surgery done because now I have all this loose skin, and I feel even worse." Plastic surgeons are great at removing the loose skin after bariatric surgery, but, sometimes, not all of it can be removed, and people must accept a certain amount of loose skin afterward no matter what. However, plastic surgery can make a huge difference. And remember, losing the excess pounds will help you live a healthier and longer life.

### Dr. Shah Recommends

If your BMI is over forty and you've tried to lose the weight on your own and just can't do it, talk to a physician who specializes in bariatric surgery.

**Options for Bariatric Surgery**

------------------------------------------------------------

If you're considering bariatric surgery, there are four major types to talk to your doctor about:

1. Lap band surgery: A plastic band is wrapped around your stomach to restrict the amount of food that is allowed into your stomach. You can lose up to 25 to 80 percent of your excess weight. Complication rate (mostly re-operation for malposition of the band) can be up to 33 percent.

2. *Roux-en-y gastric bypass surgery:* This is a procedure that combines restriction of the amount of food going to your stomach with a malabsorptive procedure that decreases the amount of calories absorbed. You can lose 50 to 70 percent of your excess weight. Complication rate can be up to 15 percent, including blood work abnormalities such as anemia due to the inability to absorb essential nutrients.

3. *Duodenal switch procedure:* This is a procedure that decreases the amount of absorption of calories by bypassing a large portion of your intestine and stomach. This is a complex procedure that requires an expert bariatric surgeon. You can lose up to 65 to 75 percent of your excess weight. The complication rate is higher (up to 24 percent), but this is because it is used most commonly for very morbidly obese people with a BMI of over fifty.

4. *The gastric sleeve:* This is the new go-to procedure for weight-loss surgery. Basically, this works by excluding a large portion of the stomach, leaving only a small "sleeve" to connect your esophagus to your intestines. The low complication rate (up to 10 percent) and great amount of weight loss (65 to 75 percent of your excess weight) has made this one of the most popular procedures for weight loss.

**Ten Psychological Reasons Some People Are Not Able to Lose Weight**

------------------------------------------------------------------

1. *Food addiction:* Food can be an addiction like cigarettes or alcohol. If you find yourself eating for no reason and you just can't stop, you should talk to a psychologist and a nutritionist about breaking this addiction cycle.

2. *Bad habits:* For example, you may have a large mocha every morning or an ice-cream sandwich before you go to bed. The best way to break a bad habit is to replace it with a good one. Have a bottle of water instead of the mocha, or cottage cheese with fruit instead of the ice cream.

3. *Eating for comfort:* We have all heard of "comfort foods" like chicken pot pie or cherry pie. Realize that these high-calorie foods can only lead to more sadness later, so go for a walk instead of opening the refrigerator.

4. *Fear of not being "socially correct":* For some reason, we all think that going out to dinner is the best way to have a social interaction. Try a bike ride or meeting for a walk. Try to not involve food in these interactions.

5. *Lack of confidence:* You think there is no way out of the hole you are in. Many people think it is impossible, or it will simply take forever to lose the excess weight. Remember that the hardest part of completing a journey is taking the first step. Start slowly and be consistent, and you will achieve your goal.

6. *Depression:* Depression causes weight gain for many reasons. If you have any of the signs of depression such as insomnia, frequent bouts of crying, or an unwillingness to be social, don't hesitate to seek help.

7. *All-or-nothing diets:* The worst diets are all-or-nothing diets that are impossible to stick to. For example, the no-carb diet is difficult to sustain for any reasonable period of time. Take small steps in the right direction, and you will do a lot better.

8. *Fasting:* You may think eating nothing all day is a good way to lose weight. Severely restricting your caloric intake puts you into starvation mode, actually making it harder to lose weight. Consult with a dietician about what is a healthy number of calories to consume daily.

9. *Sweet tooth:* There are other ways to satisfy your desire for sweets that don't involve a full portion of desert. Have a thin mint instead of a piece of chocolate cake!

10. *Lack of a plan:* Having a plan is 90 percent of the battle! Set a goal, monitor yourself daily, and give yourself feedback and reinforcement. Following this feedback loop can lead to tremendous success!

## Test Yourself

Make sure you can answer <u>yes</u> to all of these questions before you proceed.

1. Is my BMI in the normal or slightly overweight range (under thirty)?

2. Has my weight been fairly stable for the last six months (I'm not in a phase where I'm losing or gaining a lot of weight)?

3. If my BMI is over thirty, have I lost as much weight as I can, either on my own or with the aid of weight-loss surgery?

4. Have I seen before and after pictures that look like me to start with, and do I like the "afters"?

5. Am I prepared to see a gain of a few pounds immediately after my procedure due to swelling?

6. Do I have a plan to start a good exercise and diet routine after surgery (when my doctor says it is okay) so that I can continue my weight loss?

7. Have I started a diet and exercise plan now, before surgery, that I feel comfortable with?

8. Did I speak with my primary care physician regarding my weight, and has he/she tested me for other causes of weight gain (thyroid imbalance, hormone disturbances, etc.)?

9. Do I have a psychological reason for my weight being too high (food addiction, depression, etc.)?

10. Have I consulted books and websites on nutrition and healthy lifestyle so I know where to go if I have any questions, after surgery, about weight maintenance?

# Smoking

Most plastic surgeons will tell you that smoking is a deal breaker when it comes to having a cosmetic procedure. Smoking anything with nicotine slows healing tremendously and increases the risk of scarring and infection, as well as other complications. Smoking also makes the anesthesia for the surgery itself more difficult because anesthesiologists have a harder time maintaining tight control of your vitals. Postoperative pain control is also more difficult in smokers.

Although smoking is considered bad for *any* kind of plastic surgery, it is especially harmful for procedures requiring a "flap." A flap is raised when you are having a procedure involving removal of skin. Raising a flap means that we're actually lifting skin and pulling it tight and then sewing it back together. The reason this is important is because when we raise a flap, we're disconnecting blood vessels from underneath the flap so we can move the skin. When we disconnect blood vessels, we're relying on the other blood vessels that are traveling long distances to that same skin to provide healing oxygen to the tissues. It is important to know that even though the skin is the biggest organ in the body, it has some of the smallest blood vessels in the body. You can see proof of the effect of smoking on skin as smokers age. They get wrinkles a lot faster, and their skin looks thin and crepey. That's because, over many years, smoking has decreased the blood supply to the skin, and without years of adequate blood supply, the skin looks damaged and older at a much earlier age.

Patients who smoke are at an increased risk for *skin necrosis*, which is when areas of skin actually die and turn black. Necrosis of the skin (dying skin) is a difficult problem to deal with after surgery and increases the recovery time significantly. It causes scarring and infections and can, sometimes, lead to hospitalization.

Some people say, "I had gallbladder surgery, and I was smoking then, and I didn't have any problems." Gallbladder surgery is completely different from plastic surgery. The gallbladder has a huge blood supply. Skin has some of the worst blood supply of any organ in your body and is extremely vulnerable to smoking.

> **Flap Procedures**
> - - - - - - - - - - - - - - - - - - - - - - -
> Any procedure that requires a flap is particularly dangerous for smokers to undergo. Such procedures include:
>
> - tummy tuck
> - breast lift
> - face lift
> - eye lift
> - thigh lift
> - open rhinoplasty
> - back lift
> - arm lift

I sometimes hear, "I smoked after I had a C-section, and I still healed fine." Again, this is different. There is no flap of skin raised with a C-section, so you have a much better chance of healing.

## Three Scientific Reasons Why Smoking Is Bad for Wound Healing

1. The nicotine in cigarettes causes blood vessels to constrict or clamp down. That, of course, reduces the blood flow

to the skin. When you have less blood flow to the skin, less oxygen is delivered to the tissues. Without oxygen, body tissues can literally die, which is called necrosis of the tissue.

2.   When you smoke, you get carbon monoxide, not oxygen, into your lungs. The carbon monoxide is carried by your hemoglobin in place of oxygen. Hemoglobin is supposed to carry oxygen to your tissues, which is necessary for healing, but instead, in smokers, it carries carbon monoxide.

3.   When you smoke, you're also inhaling hydrogen cyanide. Hydrogen cyanide inhibits enzymes in your cells from carrying oxygen into your tissues. See the common thread here? Again, your body needs this oxygen to heal. Inhibiting the flow of oxygen to your tissue causes scarring, and, in severe cases, tissue necrosis and infection.

### Guidelines for Smokers

The best-case scenario is to quit smoking completely before you have surgery of any kind. That's the best strategy for getting you safely through surgery, the recovery process, and for your overall health. But even if you're not going to quit entirely, we tell our patients that they must give up smoking for at least four weeks before the procedure so that most of the deleterious effects of smoking have time to reverse themselves. You must also stay off cigarettes for at least four to six weeks after surgery so that your skin receives enough blood supply to heal.

After six weeks, your incisions should be healed, but if you want the scar to look its best, you should stop smoking cigarettes for the remainder of the healing process. Your scar is continually healing for up to a year or longer after surgery. Due to a lack of oxygen being delivered to the area that is healing, the scar could end up looking worse than it would have if you hadn't smoked.

Smoking before surgery is such an important issue, and the effects can be so damaging that we can't just take the patients' word that they've stayed away from cigarettes for the minimum amount of time. Unfortunately, sometimes, people will mislead their doctors so they can still have the surgery they want. In our practice, we use a urine test called the cotinine test to tell us whether there's still nicotine in a person's body. Nicotine from one cigarette can stay in the body for up to a week or longer and can be detected by this test. If a patient has a positive cotinine test, we will cancel the procedure.

### Dr. Shah Recommends

You must give up smoking for at least four weeks before your procedure and stay off cigarettes for at least six weeks after surgery. The same rules apply for marijuana, cigars, smokeless cigarettes, and nicotine patches.

### Advice on Quitting

If you're a smoker, the silver lining to all of this is that you now have a great incentive to quit in order to get the surgery you desire. I have had many patients find that their desire for a certain procedure gave them just the motivation they needed. We've seen many patients, over the years, who quit smoking to get the surgery they wanted and then stayed away from cigarettes forever! It becomes a surprise benefit, an additional cherry on top of the pie. Family members are happy, the house smells better, and the patient feels better overall. Some husbands will say to me, "I'm so glad my wife had this surgery! Not only does she look great, she's so much healthier too!"

Here are some additional tips to think about if you're considering quitting:

1.  If others in the household are smokers, encourage them to quit smoking along with you. There's a much higher chance (some studies suggest 50 percent or more) you will be successful if the other smokers in your household are not smoking and are joining you in the common goal to quit nicotine.

2.  You may want to ask your doctor for a medication such as Chantix or Zyban that can help you quit smoking. These medications do not contain nicotine and act centrally (i.e. on the brain) to decrease the craving for cigarettes.

3.  Smoking is definitely an addiction, and addictions can be effectively treated through counseling. It's a good idea to see a counselor or psychologist to help with the mental aspects of your nicotine addiction.

4.  It's okay to temporarily use nicotine patches or smokeless cigarettes to help you quit smoking, but you must also be off those for four weeks before the surgery to avoid the deleterious effects of nicotine.

5.  Different things work for different people. You have to find a way of quitting that fits into your lifestyle. Other methods for quitting that some people have used include hypnosis, acupuncture, and even over-the-counter pills that change the taste of the tobacco. There aren't many scientific studies proving these methods work, but many

people have success stories that they've been helped by these methods.

6.    Another technique you can try is called "replacement." Basically, you replace smoking with a different habit such as going for a run or eating a fruit. Some have found this technique amazingly effective.

## Dr. Shah Recommends

If you're a smoker, think about whether having this procedure could be the motivation you need to give up smoking entirely. Reward yourself for quitting by getting the procedure done after you have quit.

### Want a Face-Lift? First, Better Stop Smoking

For the last five to ten years, many plastic and cosmetic surgeons have followed my lead and refused to operate on smokers, especially those seeking a face-lift, tummy tuck, or breast-lift—procedures that require skin to be shifted.

As I shared with *New York Times* reporter Abby Ellin, the nicotine causes the tiny blood vessels in the skin to clamp down or constrict, which reduces blood supply to the skin. It can also lead to complications such as poor wound healing, increased risk of infection, longer-lasting bruises, and raised, red scars.

I certainly practice what I preached in that article, as Margaret Pyles knows firsthand. *The New York Times* featured Margaret's story prominently in the article. At the time, Margaret was a human resources director for youth homes in Bakersfield, who had come to me seeking a breast reduction. I told her that she needed to quit a minimum of thirty days before the surgery. A pack-a-day smoker since sixteen, she couldn't face battling her addiction yet again.

But once her back pain grew constant, and her abdominal muscles too flabby for her taste, Margaret came back to see me for a breast reduction, lift, tummy tuck, and liposuction—but not before she quit smoking with the help of Chantix and a hypnotist I had recommended.

She told me both helped her overcome nicotine, but fear really kept her on track. "I was afraid the anesthesia would go wrong, or I'd wake up coughing my head off and split my guts open," she said. "And I was able to stop."

The last I heard from her, Margaret had not lit up again and was thrilled that her desire to turn back the clock may also help prolong her life. "I was so focused on wanting the breast reduction more than I wanted the cigarette," she said.

Source: Abby Ellin, "Want a Face Lift? First, Better Stop Smoking," *The New York Times*, August 18, 2018, accessed January 27, 2017, http://www.nytimes.com/2008/08/14/fashion/14SKIN.html.

## Test Yourself

Carefully consider your answers to all of these questions before you proceed with surgery. If you have any risk factors, discuss them with your surgeon.

1. Do I still have nicotine in my system? (Have I smoked even a single cigarette in the last month?)

2. Have I smoked a cigar or marijuana in the last month?

3. Have I used an E-cigarette in the last month?

4. Am I prepared to stay off cigarettes and all other forms of nicotine for at least another four to six weeks following my surgery?

5. If I smoke and I am having surgery, is my surgery a "flap procedure" such as a tummy tuck, face lift, or breast lift?

6. Does someone in my family smoke inside the home and around me?

7. Does someone at my workplace smoke inside the workplace or around me?

8. Socially, will I allow others to smoke near me?

9. Is the car I use also used by a smoker?

10. Am I prepared to accept a large open wound so that I can have my surgery *and keep smoking?*

- - - - - - - - - - - - - - - - - - -

# Can't Afford to "Do It Right!"

I t is truly unfortunate to see people looking for the "best deal" they can get for their plastic surgery procedure. Radio advertisements offering unbelievable prices, Groupon deals, and "coupons" for plastic surgery are, unfortunately, everywhere now. Remember, when you purchase a procedure, what you are really "buying" is the doctor who is performing the procedure and the facility it is being performed in. Unfortunately, in the United States, any doctor can perform any kind of procedure whether or not they have been appropriately trained in that particular specialty or not. The laws really leave it up to patients to do their research on what they are paying for. Hospitals generally won't allow surgeons to do procedures that are not part of their particular specialty, but that doesn't prevent the doctor from doing it in his or her office.

There are many things to keep in mind when considering the costs of a plastic surgery procedure. In general, the total cost is usually presented as a total of multiple charges. One is the cost of the surgeon to peform the procedure itself. Then there is the cost of the operating room, which includes the sutures, gauzes, nurses, and all the supplies and people needed to perform the surgery in a safe environment. You must also factor in the cost of the anesthesiologist, who watches over you to be sure you are safely asleep for the surgery. Finally, there is the cost of any implants to be used, the cost of garments, the cost of blood work, and the cost of medications you will need after surgery. When you get a quotation for a procedure, you want all of those costs to be included in the quote and explained in detail.

There are other ancillary costs for having any type of surgery. You may have to see your primary doctor for the medical clearance that we talked about under Reason #1. If your insurance doesn't cover it, you might have to pay for it out of your own pocket. The blood work and prescriptions are often provided by a laboratory and pharmacy outside of the surgeon's practice. These additional costs must be determined as well.

Another "cost" of the procedure that you need to consider is how much income you would be losing by taking time off work or hiring additional help for yourself or for child care while you recover. You have to remember that your spouse or caretaker might need to take time off work to help you. That can reduce the household income for a little while.

Finally, there are other recovery items you might want to purchase, such as wedge pillows if you're having a tummy tuck or supportive undergarments if you're having liposuction or a breast procedure.

All of this is to say that you need to have a full and complete picture of the costs to be expected prior to signing on the dotted line. This is an important decision for you to make and one for which you do not want to cut corners.

| COSMETIC SURGICAL PROCEDURES | NATIONAL AVERAGE SURGEONS FEE |
|---|---|
| Breast augmentation (augmentation mammaplasty) | $3,543 |
| Breast implant removals (augmentation patients only) | $2,476 |
| Breast lift (mastopexy) | $4,332 |
| Breast reduction (aesthetic patients only) | $5,262 |
| Breast reduction in men (gynecomastia) | $3,194 |
| Buttock implants | $4,670 |
| Buttock lift | $4,633 |
| Calf augmentation | $3,630 |
| Cheek implant (malar augmentation) | $2,720 |
| Chin augmentation (mentoplasty) | $2,018 |
| Dermabrasion | $1,262 |
| Ear surgery (otoplasty) | $3,099 |
| Eyelid surgery (blepharoplasty) | $2,972 |
| Face lift (rhytidectomy) | $6,630 |
| Forehead lift | $3,370 |
| Hair transplantation | $5,279 |
| Lip augmentation (other than injectable materials) | $1,743 |
| Lip reduction* | $1,553 |
| Liposuction | $2,852 |
| Lower body lift | $8,082 |
| Nose reshaping (rhinoplasty) | $4,493 |
| Pectoral implants | $3,742 |
| Thigh lift | $4,756 |
| Tummy tuck (abdominoplasty) | $5,241 |
| Upper arm lift | $3,939 |

| MINIMALLY INVASIVE PROCEDURES | NATIONAL AVERAGE SURGEONS FEE |
|---|---|
| Botulinum toxin type A (Botox, Dysport) | $369 |
| Cellulite treatment (e.g., Velosmooth, Endermology) | $239 |
| Chemical peel | $712 |
| Intense pulsed light (IPL) treatment | $472 |
| Laser hair removal | $329 |
| Laser skin resurfacing | |
|     Ablative | $2,222 |
|     Nonablative (e.g., Fraxel) | $1,113 |
|     Laser treatment of leg veins | $364 |
|     Microdermabrasion | $154 |
|     Sclerotherapy | $351 |
| Soft tissue fillers | |
|     Calcium hydroxylapatite (e.g., Radiesse) | $631 |
|     Collagen | |
|     Porcine/bovine based (e.g., Evolence, Zyderm, Zyplast) | $428 |
|     Human based (e.g., Cosmoderm, Cosmoplast, Cymetra) | $529 |
| Fat | $1,604 |
| Hyaluronic acid (e.g., Juvederm Ultra, Juvederm Ultra Plus, Perlane, Prevelle Silk, Restylane) | $538 |
| Polylactic acid (Sculptra) | $908 |
| Polymethyl-methacrylate microspheres (Artefill) | $1,065 |

*Data from the American Society of Plastic Surgeons: 2012 Plastic Surgery Statistics Report.

## Beware of the "Cut-Rate" Solution

This chart of basic costs will give you an idea of what doctors charge, on average, for various procedures. What is presented here is a national average, so you'll have to take into account the average costs in your local market. Another reason I included these costs is so that you can compare them with your doctor's quotation. Your par- ticular quote might be slightly higher or lower, but a warning sign is if something is much lower than the average. There are a lot of people doing cosmetic surgery today, especially in the United States, who have not been trained appropriately. Many have learned how to do these types of procedure over a weekend course! Weekend courses do not train doctors to do these procedures correctly or handle the complications that might occur afterward. So if your doctor's quote is significantly cheaper than what you see here, you're going to want to ask why. Just as with anything else, if the price sounds too good to be true, there's usually a (bad) reason behind it.

You also want to be suspicious of doctors who are performing major surgeries under local anesthesia in their office. The reason why some doctors perform major procedures such as breast aug- mentations or tummy tucks under local anesthesia is that they are not allowed to do these procedures at a hospital or a surgery center because they're not able to obtain credentials to do so. Doctors who are not real plastic surgeons usually cannot get privileges at surgery centers and hospitals. So again, if a doctor is doing an actual surgery at a medspa or in the back room of an office, that's very suspect. It's really important that your surgical procedure is treated like any other surgery because the complications could be just as real.

A great question to ask is, "Do you have privileges to perform these procedures at a local hospital?" Knowing that a doctor has hospital privileges gives you a better idea of how well trained and established your doctor is. A hospital will usually not give privileges to doctors who have not been adequately trained in the procedure they are going to perform.

Another great question is, "Did you complete a plastic surgery fellowship program?" This will tell you whether the doctor completed the necessary additional training in plastic surgery to become board certified.

Watch out for practices who advertise lots of discounts. Plastic surgery is not like going to a hair salon where you can take in a coupon and get a cheaper price. Whenever physicians are "cheapening" something, you have to wonder where they're cutting corners and how vested they are in getting a good result.

Cutting corners is also a sign of lack of quality and care. It saves you some money if they don't have to hire an anesthesiologist, for example. But using local anesthesia for major procedures creates the risk of lidocaine overdose, not to mention pain and discomfort during the procedure. The procedure usually takes a lot longer under local anesthesia. Also the local anesthesia can wear off during the surgery. This can result in surgical errors while trying to perform a precise procedure because the patient has become a "moving target."

The facility where you have your surgery should be either a hospital or a certified surgery center. Outpatient surgery centers are certified by a few different accreditation bodies. These include JCAHO, AAAASF, AAAHC, and the State. Always ask if the procedure you are having is going to take place in a "certified surgery center" or hospital.

It's a good idea to visit a few doctors to find one who is properly qualified, one with the education and experience that will increase your chances of great results. Choose a doctor you trust, one with whom you have a great connection. Surgery, plastic or otherwise, is not a field where it makes a lot of sense to go around price shopping. It's your life and your well-being at stake. The major downside of opting for a cheap and easy solution is that the procedure is less likely to turn out the way you want. The doctor likely won't have the right resources on hand to deal with complications if you're in the back room of an office. Patients have been known to die in such instances. There are tons of reports in the news about non-plastic surgeons performing plastic surgery in the back room of an office and their patient actually dying during or after the procedure because the staff and the doctor had no idea how to handle the complication. In general, plastic surgery is extremely safe when done by a well-trained surgeon in the correct setting. But having a doctor who took a weekend course on performing your plastic surgery is like getting in a car with a ten-year-old child and asking him/her to drive you from New York City to New Jersey. It's just not a smart thing to do.

### Buying Time for Recovery

Another aspect of the overall costs of your procedure is the recovery. Be sure that you have the resources, in terms of both finances and time, to recover properly. You should not go back to work before you've recovered or try to do things such as lifting the kids before your wounds have healed. These activities will not only risk your health, but you also risk undoing the desired effects of the surgery you just went through. Wounds might not heal as well or as fast, there might be scarring, or you might have to go back to surgery because you ripped your stitches or encountered some other complication. No one who has plastic surgery wants an outcome like that, so you have to make sure you budget for a proper recovery. That can mean taking time off work and, perhaps, hiring extra help to take over your household responsibilities while you heal. (More on this subject in Reason #8: You Don't Have the Time, and Reason #9: You Don't Have the Support System.)

## The Reality of Botched Procedures

I get many patients who say they have had their procedure "botched" by another doctor and they want me to correct it. I usually find that this term is used quite loosely, and often incorrectly, by most patients. There could be complications that occur with any procedure that are not the fault of the surgeon performing the procedure. Also, many people say they are "botched" when it is really just seeing something that is part of their anatomy normally. In any case, the reality is that if you have a reputable plastic surgeon performing your surgery, you will be warned of these issues before you undergo the surgery so you can be prepared.

Always consider the cost to you if things go wrong. You may have to pay for an unexpected stay in the hospital, recovery costs, and having the surgery done all over again. With plastic surgery, you really only have one chance to do it right. Fixing it can end up costing you a lot more money and a lot more problems later on. You might not ever be able to get it fixed correctly. Plastic surgery is definitely one area in which you want to spend the money upfront to get it right the first time rather than end up chasing your tail and "hoping for the best" with the cheap procedure.

It is important to understand is that any sort of complication just costs you more in the long run and can also lead to an unhappy result. Remember that the fewer times the surgeon has to operate, the fewer times the surgeon raises a flap of skin, the better. The more times a particular procedure is done in the same location (known as a revision), the harder it is for the body to heal and the more scar tissue there's going to be. Scar tissue is never as good as real tissue. It's harder. It has less blood supply. It doesn't look as good. The more often scar tissue is cut, the less well it heals, and eventually it may not heal at all. You want to give yourself every opportunity to get it right the first time by investing in the right doctor, by taking enough time off, and by investing in whatever else you need to help you recover fully. Plastic surgery is truly an area where an up-front investment pays off in the long run.

## Test Yourself

Make sure you can answer <u>yes</u> to all of these questions before you proceed.

1. Is your doctor allowed to perform these procedures at a local hospital?

2. Is the procedure being performed at an accredited surgery center or a hospital (not a room in the office)?

3. Did your doctor do a fellowship in plastic surgery allowing him/her to become board certified in plastic surgery? (This training program takes two years or more; a weekend course does not count.)

4. Have you asked your doctor, "How many of these procedures have you done and for how long have you been performing them?"

5. Have you asked your doctor, "Have your patients suffered any serious complications?"

6. Have you viewed the doctor's before and after pictures on his website?

7. Have you researched the doctor's credentials, and do you feel comfortable with them?

8. Do you have a full picture of the costs associated with the procedure, including the physician's fee, fees from the hospital and anesthesiologist, the cost of taking time off work and getting the help you need, as well as any other ancillary costs?

9. Can you comfortably afford the cost without being tempted to cut corners?

- - - - - - - - - - - - - - - - - -

# Wanting Surgery for the Wrong Reasons

P lastic surgeons frequently are asked to consult with people who have an objective in mind that cannot be achieved. For this reason, we constantly find ourselves in the position of having to protect the patients from themselves. Here are some of the common ones that people struggle with:

### "I Want to Look Like a Celebrity"

Referring to what you conceive as a result that you would like to aim for by sharing a celebrity picture with your surgeon is sometimes helpful. We often hear, "I want Angelina Jolie's lips," or "Beyonce's butt," which, in and of itself, is fine. Pictures can give your doctor a point of reference that can be very helpful in discussing your options. But you have to believe your doctor if he/she tells you that you won't achieve the result you're hoping for and what you are requesting is not realistic. People sometimes have the misconception that if they can make themselves look like a celebrity, they'll suddenly have the lifestyle celebrities possess. That is, of course, unrealistic thinking, but some people truly believe (often subconsciously) this is true. Bringing in a picture of a celebrity and saying, "I don't care what it takes; make me look exactly like Justin Bieber," is a huge red flag to plastic surgeons. Plastic surgery is not able to completely change the way you look into the exact replica of another person. We can only make subtle changes that refine or contour specific areas. A completely new look is not only rarely possible but also dangerous. Too much surgery on your face can cause complications and an overall "fake" look.

Again, it's not illegal for doctors to do any procedure you request, so you have to look out for yourself. You want to be wary of any surgeon who declares, "Yes, I can make you look like that celebrity!" That is a false promise and doomed for disappointment.

### "I Want the Latest Surgery Fad"

Another reason I often counsel patients in their choice to perform a procedure is a concern that they are following a fad. It's common nowadays to hear, all of a sudden, something become the topic of discussion in the media or in magazines such as *Us Weekly*. Again, a couple of perfect examples are Angelina Jolie's lips and Beyonce's buttocks. Often, new laser procedures make use of a large marketing budget; advertisers spend millions of dollars to get popular television shows to generate "buzz" over the course of a few months.

Having large lips like Angelina Jolie doesn't look right on most people's faces. Beyonce's butt might not fit your body type or your lifestyle. And even if it is possible for you to have a butt similar to Beyonce's, just because she's popular today doesn't mean it's necessarily right for you over the long term. Many laser devices or technologies are often launched without long-term patient experience proving effectiveness in a majority of the patients. Remember, you can't change your body with the seasons the way you do your clothes. Your body doesn't heal well after multiple surgeries on the same body part. You might like something now but not down the road, and having the procedure reversed will be difficult later on. You should think about what you want your body or face to look like *over time*, not just right now. How will this procedure look on you ten, twenty, or thirty years from now? With plastic surgery, most of the time, it is impossible to "go back" and take away the effects of a procedure. So be careful when following the latest plastic surgery trends.

### "Someone Caused Me to Lose Self-Esteem, and I'm Trying to Get It Back"

Almost every day, people come to our office because their significant other, spouse, or even a "friend" has poked fun of or drawn attention to a certain part of their body and made them feel as though it looks "terrible " or "unsightly." These nasty comments make these people feel depressed and extremely self-conscious.

Don't change something about your body just because someone says something negative about you. You want to make sure you make changes for yourself, not because someone made you self-conscious. Many times, the motivation of the person putting you down is misguided and may come from jealousy, envy, or their own insecurity. That person may be manipulating you by tearing down your self-esteem. Remind yourself that those who make negative comments about your body, especially if you didn't invite these comments, are just rude and tactless.

By the same token, if you have just been forced to end a relationship with a significant other, changing the way you look absolutely doesn't mean you're going to get that person back in your life. Unfortunately, we encounter this misconception all too often in this profession.

"My husband just left me for a younger woman! I want you to make me look young and hot again so I can get him back." That request almost always leads to disappointment and regret. And do you really want a person in your life that would return for physical reasons? Reputable physicians will probably suggest that those individuals take a six-month pause and come back after that if they still want the procedure. Or they might suggest talking to a psychologist or a relationship advisor about the issue. It's really important that you are in the right "place" in life to have cosmetic surgery. "Bounce-back" surgery is rarely a good idea.

## "I'm in a Bad Place in My Life, and I Want the Surgery so I'll Feel Better"

If you are currently involved in any kind of crisis, now is not the right time for plastic surgery. Examples of crisis situations which should cause pause are a death in the family, loss of a job, midlife crisis, or bullying at work or at school. Crisis situations are usually psychological minefields that are difficult for anyone to navigate and usually involve emotions that change from minute to minute. If you are going through any kind of crisis, you should really work through the situation (often, simply letting time pass is the ultimate crisis resolution plan) before undergoing surgery, with the full understanding that surgery itself is not going to end the crisis. More often than not, people don't get their job back because they've had plastic surgery, and surgery won't make it any easier to recover from a loss. You want to avoid making a big decision like this when you're in some sort of panicked or emotional state. If you're in a state of crisis, you can actually make things worse by relying on plastic surgery to solve issues for you that it just can't solve. Moreover, stress has profound effects on your ability to heal, so surgery in mid-crisis is not the right time anyway. You want to be in a state of calm when you do this, in order to optimize your ability to heal well.

All of this doesn't mean that life has to be perfect before you have plastic surgery. Who has a perfect life all the time? Now, if you've already been through a situation like a divorce, for instance, and you are some distance from it, that's a different situation. A procedure can be a huge confidence booster for people in situations like that who are trying to get their lives back on track. The self-esteem boost from looking your best cannot be denied, but it needs to be timed well, during a period of emotional and life stability.

The smart patient usually come in because they're unhappy with some physical aspect of themselves. They've considered the pros and cons for some time, talked to their trusted advisors and loved ones about their decision, and

## Choosing Not to Have Surgery

I once saw a patient who was an overweight college kid and he was getting bullied at school. The bullying was so bad that he had actually tried to commit suicide. His parents brought him in because they thought the only way to help him and to keep him in school was for him to get liposuction.

I wanted to help, but I had to say to them, "It sounds like there are a lot of things going on here, and plastic surgery, especially liposuction, is not going to cure all the issues." I talked them out of having him undergo the surgery, and instead, we came up with a multipronged approach to help him solve his problems. One was to talk to the counselors at school. Another was to get him psychological help for the suicide attempt. And finally, we put him in a weight loss and exercise program. Liposuction was never going to be able to do all those things for him.

arrived at a point where they believe plastic surgery can really help them feel better about themselves. Research has shown, as has my personal experience, that plastic surgery can make a large improvement in a person's life, self-confidence, and self-worth. It can truly add a "spring" to your step!

### Test Yourself

Make sure you can answer <u>yes</u> to all of these questions before you proceed.

1. Do you understand that plastic surgery can't make you look completely like someone else?

2. Do you know that plastic surgery will not get you the lifestyle of anyone you are trying to look like?

3. Have you thought about whether this is a change you're going to want over the long term and not just because it's what's in fashion right now?

4. Are you giving in to a "fad" in the media without really checking out the reality and potential risks of the procedure?

5. Are you doing this for yourself and not for someone else?

6. Are you sure that you are not undergoing surgery because someone said something to you that hurt your feelings and made you self-conscious?

7. Are you past any crisis points in your life and making the decision with a clear head?

- - - - - - - - - - - - - - - - - - -

# Unrealistic Expectations

B eing realistic about your outcome is a high-priority conversation you should always have with your plastic surgeon. It is of utmost importance for a patient to understand what surgery is capable of changing and to what degree. If you expect something that is impossible to achieve, you are setting yourself up for failure.

The results that can be obtained are going to be different from patient to patient. Although we generally encourage our patients to look through before and after pictures in the office or on the Internet, it's important to remember that finding an after picture you like doesn't mean we can create that same result for you. I sometimes explain it to my patients with this analogy: Plastic surgery is not like shopping in a catalog for a coat. If you want a fur coat, but the catalog only has wool, you aren't going to get a fur coat, no matter what. When looking through before and after pictures, find before pictures of people who looked the way you look now and look at those patients' after-surgery results. Then pick the ones you like. Don't find a before picture that looks nothing like you and expect the after results to be realistic for you. All too often we see people coming in with pictures of bikini models when they themselves are forty pounds overweight. Without a total change in your lifestyle, over many years, a change that drastic cannot be achieved with plastic surgery.

Here are some signs that your expectations aren't as reasonable as they need to be:

## You Want to Look Like a Celebrity (or Exactly Like Someone Else)

Plastic surgery cannot radically change your bone structure, skin, muscle, or fat so much that you will look exactly like another person or even give you any of that person's exact physical characteristics. Often we encounter patients who have the misguided notion that *looking like someone else* is going to give the lifestyle of that person. There is no way that looking like a celebrity is going to give you the attention or opportunities that someone else has. Too often, we see people who say they want to look like Brad Pitt, J. Lo, or Kim Kardashian. Although it is okay to refer to the type of result you want ("I want Angelina Jolie-type lips"), you need to know that you will not suddenly be transported to a mansion in Beverly Hills and make movies. You also need to know that Angelina Jolie's lips look good on Angelina Jolie, J. Lo's buttocks look good on J. Lo, and so on. This type of result may not look good on you because the rest of "you" is completely different.

## You Want the Results to Turn Out Perfect

As doctors, we watch out for people who are trying to achieve perfection, because we know there's no such thing. Even when you're born, you're not perfect. Everyone is asymmetric to some degree. All of us have small flaws or variations in our skin. People who are obsessed with their version of perfection are a red flag to doctors, often signaling they have obsessive-compulsive disorder. If you really take a close look at people who look "perfect," you will see many imperfections. Next time you get a chance, take a close look at a picture of your favorite "perfect-looking" model or celebrity without makeup (search #nomakeup on Instagram), and you'll see what I mean. Our beauty actually lies in our imperfections, the small asymmetries or marks that draw our eye into the person's soul (Joaquin Phoenix's lip or Marilyn Monroe's mole are perfect examples.) A slight asymmetry or mark is not only "normal" but desirable for a natural look.

### You're Impossible to Please

Another type of patient whom surgeons watch out for is someone who's impossible to please. They are often people who talk to the doctor for a long time and ask the same questions over and over again because they're seeking the answers they want, not the ones they're hearing. There are some people who are just not going to be happy with the results, no matter what you tell them or how well the procedure goes.

If you feel you're not getting the answers you want, even after seeing many doctors, you might fall into this category. If that's the case, you might want to look into the deeper reason behind what you're seeking. If you see ten doctors, and nine of them recommend the same thing, and one says he can do what you want him to do, that also should be a red flag to you. In general, if you're seeing qualified doctors, and all but one of them is recommending the same thing, that one doctor is probably just telling you what you want to hear (or has a mortgage payment due). But it's unlikely that he/she will be able to live up to what's being promised.

### You're Obsessed with a Minor Defect

Something that's so minor that you're measuring it with a ruler is not going to be easily corrected with plastic surgery. Say, for example, one eyebrow is just a millimeter higher than the other, or your nose is one millimeter off-center—so slightly off center that only you notice it when you're looking very closely in a mirror. Maybe the nipple on your right breast is shaped just a little differently than the one on your left breast. These things are normal. Everyone has some degree of "normal" differences from one side to the other, and it's not realistic to expect to obtain a totally symmetrical degree of perfection. Plastic surgery is an art, and the body is a constantly changing, unpredictable canvas. It's not like building a desk, for which you can measure something down to the millimeter and shave it off. Your body will change as it's healing. Gravity, swelling, and overall health all affect your healing process. Scar tissue, genetics, and forces of nature are involved. These are all, by and large, totally unpredictable. Even though plastic surgeons can make things a lot better, it doesn't mean you should try to correct every minor defect. If your doctor tells you that it's a minor problem not worth correcting, you should really think twice and consider what he/she said. If you are still bothered by it, you should get a second opinion. If you get the same opinion again, you may want to rethink the issue.

### You Expect Perfect Symmetry

Any part of the body that has "two sides"—the eyes, the eyebrows, and particularly, the breasts—are areas where some people get hung up on the idea that the two sides should be exactly alike. But that's just not the way any of us are made. To expect perfect symmetry is unrealistic, and perfect symmetry can even make you look unnatural.

I remember a very powerful exercise I went through in my plastic surgery training (see the following example). We were asked to take a photo of someone's face, create a mirror image of the left side, and put that mirror image on the right side so that the face appeared exactly symmetrical. We did the same for the right half of the face. The results were astonishing. The photos appeared to be of two completely different people, neither of whom looked anything like the original person! Quite frankly, the "perfect symmetry" photos looked odd. Asymmetry is completely normal, and it's impossible to expect perfect symmetry from surgery. Your surgeon might be able to match things more closely but not perfectly. You should know this before you discuss your expectations with your doctor.

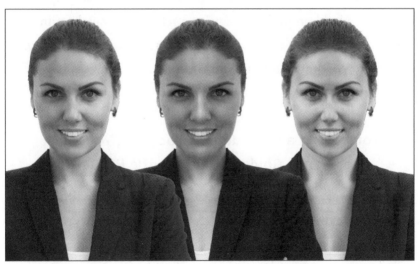

**NORMAL**          **LEFT**          **RIGHT**

## You Want to Lose a *Lot* of Weight

Overweight people who think a surgery such as liposuction or a tummy tuck is going to help them lose a lot of weight on the scale are going to be extremely disappointed. You may actually only lose a few pounds with liposuction or a tummy tuck. Liposuction and tummy tuck procedures are great for contouring the body and taking care of problem areas, often making you *look* as if you've lost twenty pounds or more. However, on the scale, you may only see the loss of two or three pounds on average and almost surely less than five. That amount of weight loss is not going to turn you into a thin person if you're not one to begin with. If you are looking for weight loss, the only solution is to hit the gym and eat a balanced diet.

I often have patients who come back for their first postoperative visit (a few days after surgery) surprised and depressed that they have gained weight. I explain to them that the trauma of surgery causes the body to hold on to fluids, causing swelling and weight gain. This process takes a full a month or longer to reverse itself. It may take months to see any significant weight loss, and that occurs only in combination with exercise and diet.

## You've Had a Procedure Already, but You Think the Results Could Be Just a Little Bit Better

The enemy of "good" in plastic surgery is "better." Think about Michael Jackson's nose. That was a case where trying to change too much or make it look too perfect led to something that looked worse and worse over time, much worse than it did to begin with. Michael Jackson underwent many plastic surgery procedures to change minor problems. As I've said before, too much surgery can be a big problem. Good plastic surgeons take the time to get it right the first time because every subsequent procedure can lead to a higher rate of complication and dissatisfaction. You should be happy with the results if they are pretty close to what you wanted because trying to revise a surgery over and over again just to make it "a little bit better" is usually a good way to end up with a complication.

Revisions (or touch ups) should never be rushed into. In my opinion, you should always wait at least six months to a year between surgeries. The body has a tremendous ability to "shape" itself over time, obviating the need for a revision surgery. Rushing back into the operating room is never a good idea.

## You Want the Change to Last Forever

Liposuction can help you trim a problem area such as love handles or belly fat, but the effects aren't going to last forever if you eat a double cheeseburger every day for lunch and dinner. You can have a procedure to help the appearance of your skin, but the effect is not going to last all that long if you continue to smoke or spend time in the sun. Your results will last even less time if you don't take care of yourself during recovery and beyond. Even when you do take good care of yourself, the body is constantly changing (and, yes, aging). Gravity and the aging process will continue to affect the way you look forever. Gravity and time affect some people more than others, depending on your genetics and skin elasticity. No matter what, your breast lift or augmentation will sag over time (this effect is reduced by wearing a bra as much as possible), your face lift will wrinkle with time, and your liposuction areas will get larger with weight gain.

Hopefully, you have a good doctor who is giving you a realistic picture so you will be happy with the result. But if your doctor is promising you the moon and saying the results of your procedure will last forever, that should be a warning that perhaps your doctor isn't someone you should trust.

- - - - - - - - - - - - - - - - -

# Unresolved Psychological Challenges

Anyone who has a current, untreated psychological diagnosis is not a candidate for plastic surgery. That doesn't mean that if a person does have a diagnosis, they can not have surgery ever, but they should be being treated for the disorder and they should discuss the idea of having plastic surgery at length with their psychologist first. Make sure your psychologist is involved in the entire process of the procedure—before, during, and after. You may need a dosage adjustment of any medications, as well as counseling through the different stages of recovery.

The reason why this is so important is that plastic surgery has been shown to magnify certain psychological ailments. After surgery, people are more likely to feel scared and vulnerable. They can't move around as much. They're stuck at home recovering. They're in some degree of pain, which can cause changes in the hormonal activity of your body and brain. Having surgery releases stress hormones from the adrenal glands that affect your mood and thinking. All these drastic hormonal changes can be tough for anyone to deal with, but they can be even harder on people with a psychiatric diagnosis. This means that if you have obsessive-compulsive disorder (OCD), depression, or anxiety, and it's not under control when you have the procedure done, then you can have significant problems and worsening symptoms in the immediate postoperative period. Even if your disorder is under control, your symptoms may be magnified, which is why it's important that your psychologist be involved every step of the way.

## Body Dysmorphic Disorder

Body dysmorphic disorder is a serious psychiatric diagnosis. People affected by this disorder are extremely preoccupied with their own minor or imaginary physical flaws. When people with body dysmorphic disorder look in the mirror, they see someone who is completely different from themselves. They may be overly focused on their skin, their hair, or their nose. They may be excessively focused on facial lines and tiny marks on their face. They constantly think of themselves as fat, despite being thin or normal weight. (Sometimes this disorder can lead to anorexia or bulimia.) They spend a lot of time looking in the mirror and trying to hide their perceived imperfections. They might also spend a lot of time talking about those imperfections and comparing them to the way others look. They may spend a lot of time seeking reassurance from others about how they look. These are all symptoms of body dysmorphic disorder.

People with this disorder often seek out plastic surgery, but the big problem is that they will almost surely feel worse after having the procedure. They will never be happy with the outcome of the surgery because of their disorder. They may think that the way to feel better is to fix the flaw they're focused on, but what they really need is a cognitive behavioral therapist who can provide counseling and possible medications such as SSRIs or antidepressants.

## Other Disorders

Surgery is a stressful event and a psychologically intense experience. Everything is magnified because not only do you have the normal anxieties and stresses about having surgery, you're also putting your hopes and expectations for an improved image and lifestyle on top of that. More than any other kind of surgery, plastic surgery creates a particular and more intense risk of psychological issues revealing themselves.

The following is a list of some additional disorders which you should consult your psychologist about prior to having plastic surgery. If you've been diagnosed with one of these disorders, or suspect you might suffer from any one of them, it is important to seek psychiatric help. This is not a complete list, so talk to your doctor or psychologist about any issues that might be of concern to you.

- depression
- substance abuse
- any type of social phobia
- any eating disorder
- obsessive-compulsive disorder (OCD)
- any type of anxiety disorder
- attention deficit disorder
- bulimia
- anorexia

## Prepare Yourself Psychologically

Cosmetic surgery can be a major life-changing experience. You will be riding an emotional roller coaster on which you may experience

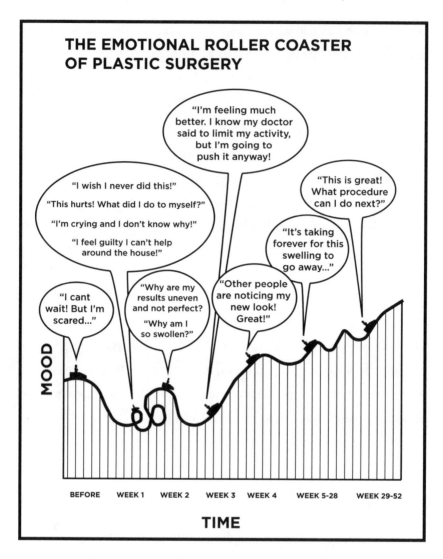

depression, frustration, and excitement. So it's important to be well prepared psychologically for this experience. To help you prepare, do the following:

1. Fill out the following psychological questionnaire, and bring it to your preoperative appointment.

2. Talk with your family and close friends you trust about what you will be going through. Remind them it is important to be positive and supportive during your healing process,

and if you do get depressed or "weird" after surgery, they should tell your doctor on your behalf.

3. Feel comfortable in letting the doctor know if you are experiencing any postoperative depression or other feelings that are not normal for you. Your doctor has many temporary remedies for these issues.

# PSYCHOLOGICAL QUESTIONNAIRE

Please list your previous cosmetic surgeries

| TYPE | DATE | SURGEON | SATISFIED with OUTCOME? |
|------|------|---------|------------------------|
|  |  |  | YES  NO |
|  |  |  | YES  NO |
|  |  |  | YES  NO |
|  |  |  | YES  NO |
|  |  |  | YES  NO |

Have you been compliant with all recent medical treatment recommended/prescribed by your physician and/or OB/GYN?      Y      N

Do you have sudden mood swings (from feeling okay to being enraged)?      Y      N

Do you have a pattern of intense, unstable personal relationships?      Y      N

Have you ever deliberately hurt yourself physically?      Y      N

Have you ever attempted suicide?      Y      N

Have you felt depressed within the last year?      Y      N

Do you cry for no apparent reason?      Y      N

Have you felt that your weight or appearance has been the cause of failures in life?      Y      N

Do you frequently worry about your appearance?      Y      N

Do you frequently compare your appearance to others?      Y      N

Are you very concerned about the appearance of some part of your body that you consider flawed or unattractive?      Y      N

Do people frequently disagree with your opinion of your perceived body flaw?      Y      N

Do you frequently check your appearance in mirrors?      Y      N

Do you feel that your life is compromised by your concerns with your appearance?      Y      N

Is your significant other supportive of your decision to have plastic surgery?      Y      N

Do you feel that this procedure should
totally change your life?                                    Y        N

Does your weight fluctuate more than
ten pounds every few months?                                 Y        N

Do you think that you will look perfect
after having this procedure?                                 Y        N

Are you currently going through a divorce or having major
problems in your relationship with your significant other?   Y        N

Have you ever been anorexic or bulimic?                      Y        N

Have you ever used illegal street drugs or prescription drugs?   Y    N

List all your psychological diagnoses (current and past):

_____

_____

## Test Yourself

Make sure you can answer <u>yes </u>to all of these questions before you
proceed.

1.  Are you in good psychological health?

2.  If you've received a diagnosis of any of the disorders mentioned
    in this section, have you talked with your psychologist about
    your plans to have plastic surgery?

3.  If you've received a diagnosis of any of the disorders mentioned
    in this section, have you informed your plastic surgeon about
    that diagnosis?

4.  Have you filled out the above psychiatric history form and
    given it to your doctor?

5.  Have you talked to your trusted family members and friends
    who know about your planned surgery and asked for their
    support during the healing process?

6.  Do you accept the fact that you may experience temporary
    mood swings, depression, and other feelings after your surgery
    and that you should talk to your surgeon about them?

7.  Have you mentally prepared yourself for the healing process,
    sometimes up to a year, needed to obtain your results?

------------------------------------

# Lack of Time

A common misconception is that since plastic surgery is usually performed as an outpatient procedure, that it is as easy as going to a hair stylist for a new hair-do. The portrayal of an entire plastic surgery journey in thirty-minute programs on cable television has lead to many having a severely skewed view of how much time goes into deciding, researching, and recovering from plastic surgery. Often six to eight weeks of recovery time are skipped over in the blink of an eye, often during a commercial break.

Also, keep in mind when you talk to others who have already had surgery that people also tend to forget uncomfortable moments, especially those times when they were immediately post-op on pain medications. You may hear, "It was no big deal. I recovered fast," which does not realistically communicate how much time it actually took to recover.

It's a lot like giving birth: mothers often only remember the good parts of their time having a baby, and the painful delivery is rarely ever a topic of conversation  In addition, memory can't always be trusted.

People's lives seem to be getting busier and busier. Often the time period of the surgery fades away, and people forget the time they invested into it. Many of us juggle all sorts of things at once, including work, kids, the responsibilities of the household, and so on. Sound like you? Too many people don't understand that when you have any kind of surgical procedure, not just plastic surgery, you really should plan your life around the surgery and not try to wedge the surgery into your life. That means more than just planning to take a day or two off to have the procedure. You also want to plan for enough time to have a good recovery. It is not easy to recover from a surgical procedure. There's a lot you must factor in, including not just your physical recovery but also your mental recovery.

## Time for Your Physical Recovery

Most plastic surgery procedures are not something your body can recover from overnight. There will be a few days that you are barely, to move around to take care of yourself. You may not be able to climb stairs or even get out of bed without help. For a few days after surgery, you will feel totally incapacitated. Do not plan to go out of town for a vacation, go to family events, a work party, or anything of the sort for at least two to six weeks after your procedure. (Ask your doctor what he/she recommends.) All too often we see serious complications in the healing of patients who use their two-week vacation to have a breast augmentation and go to Florida for spring break. That is a disaster waiting to happen.

My best advice is to overprepare for your recovery. Set yourself up in the most comfortable place you can think of to recover. That's almost always your home, your mom's home, or a recovery center where the staff specialize in plastic surgery recovery. Take a little bit too much time off, think of everything possible you may need, have too much help around, and read everything your doctor gives you three times.

What could happen if you rush yourself and get back to normal life too soon? Some common complications of overdoing it after surgery include fainting and hurting yourself, bleeding from your incisions or inside your body (a hematoma), slow healing, open wounds, infections, and hospitalization. Doesn't sound like fun, does it? In fact, you could add months to your recovery time by causing a complication, and you could permanently ruin your results. What a waste of time, money, and energy just so you could go to the office holiday party the week after your tummy tuck. It's not worth it, in my opinion.

Here are a few additional words of caution. Are you one of those people who "heal quickly" from surgery? Do you "barely feel pain" or start doing housework the day after surgery? Your pain medication can trick you into believing that you have healed because you feel minimal pain. Don't fool yourself and believe you have some superhuman capacity to heal. Remember that your memory (and your pain level) can trick you! Don't try to be the tough guy or gal, because the results can be disastrous.

Before you sign on the dotted line, you need to be thinking about time away from work. In general, if you have a desk job, you'll have to take off a week to two weeks (ask your surgeon). If you do anything physical in your job, including having to walk around a lot, recovery could take six weeks to three months.

These same guidelines apply to stay-at-home moms. Parenting is hard work, so you need one to two weeks of recovery time, at minimum, before you can resume your parenting responsibilities. And if your kids are at an age that necessitates a lot of physical activity, such as frequently driving them around or lifting a child who weighs twenty pounds or more, then you must give yourself longer. Often, I tell my patients it's time for grandma to move in or for the husband to take a few weeks off. Don't underestimate your healing time. Plastic surgery is real surgery, and your body needs adequate time to heal.

An additional note on facial plastic surgery: If you don't want to tell your colleagues at work that you've had a procedure done, then you need to think about budgeting time not just to feel better but also for all the telltale signs to disappear. You should plan on not looking "healed" for at least three to four weeks and possibly longer.

## Time for Your Mental Recovery

It's important to note that it will take some time before you feel like yourself again after surgery. Having a cosmetic procedure done is unlike any other surgical experience. For reasons that we can only guess, cosmetic surgery causes a roller coaster of emotional experiences in the immediate postoperative period. So many of our hopes, desires, and expectations are associated with the way we feel about our looks, so plastic surgery can cause emotional turmoil as we go through the stages of healing.

For example, many people report a feeling of depression after surgery. Sometimes, patients come into my office and tell me they're crying every day and don't know why. They say they are happy with how everything is going, but their brain is stuck in an emotional state that they cannot shake.

The depression, anxiety, restlessness, and other feelings that many patients experience don't necessarily have anything to do with the plastic surgery itself. After every surgical procedure, you are going to experience huge changes in activity and lifestyle, especially for the first few weeks. One day you're running around and doing all sorts of things, and the next, you're mostly confined to your bed. When you can't do the things you want and end up spending a lot of time in one place, it can lead to depression.

There's another emotion that creeps its way into patients' minds and can lead to the depression people experience after surgery. That emotion is guilt. Many people feel guilty about temporarily shirking their responsibilities to their family, their kids, and their job in order to have an elective procedure. They feel they're putting other people out. Between feeling guilty and being unable to move around and do the things you normally do, you sometimes go through a downward spiral of emotions until you end up crying and feeling sad for reasons you can't explain.

The postoperative depression stage might be followed by a feeling some describe simply as craziness. Your emotions are up, your emotions are down, and you don't know what to think or how to react. In our practice we call this the "erratic period." Major hormonal changes occur after surgery. Remember that your body doesn't know the difference between a surgical procedure and being hit by a truck. Your stress hormones act as though you got into a major accident, and your body does what it is genetically programmed to do, which is to go into a "shock" state. You have a huge outpouring of stress hormones from the glands in your brain. When this abrupt rise in stress hormones dissipates, your body realizes it is going to be okay, and you almost go into a "downward" effect, similar to coming off a drug. These hormone changes that all people experience after surgery is a big reason that you end up having psychological experiences that you have never felt before.

Things start normalizing about two to four weeks after surgery, depending on what type of procedure you had done. It could be four to six weeks before you really feel like yourself again. These kinds of changes in mood are something you need to watch out for during recovery time. You need to plan sufficient time for this kind of recovery, and that requires having a conversation with your caretakers, family, and friends before your surgery to make sure they have a good understanding of how to help you through the recovery period.

## Your First Forty-Eight Hours after Surgery

We give all our patients the following instructions after surgery. Read through them to get a better idea of what to expect. These are meant to be guidelines for discussion only. Please check with your surgeon on his/her specific instructions to follow:

*Very important: If you have excessive bleeding or pain, call your doctor immediately.*

*Caretaker: If you are going home, a family member or friend who is at least eighteen years of age must drive you home, and that person should stay overnight with you. It is preferred that someone be with you to help you at all times after surgery, for at least three to four days. Also, since you are sedated and have limited mobility, this person should be able to help you get in and out of bed and help you to go to the bathroom. It should, of course, be someone you are comfortable with. If you choose to go to a postoperative center, they will provide transportation. If you have any questions about these matters, please ask one of our nursing staff.*

*Dressings: Keep your dressings as clean and dry as possible for the first thirty-six hours (one and a half days). After this time you may remove all the dressings and any garments you are wearing. Keep the Steri-Strips (clear white tape) or the skin glue on the incisions undisturbed. You may shower thirty-six hours (one and a half days) after surgery. It is okay to get the incisions wet after thirty-six hours. You may reapply any surgical garments after your shower. You should consider having help for your shower, as many people do feel faint during their first shower. Also, consider sitting on a plastic stool while showering.*

*Activity: Take it easy and pamper yourself for at least two weeks after surgery. Avoid any and all straining and do not lift anything heavier than a gallon of milk. If something hurts at all, stop the activity. If you feel tired, immediately rest. You may go to the bathroom, sit and watch TV, read some books, walk to the kitchen table for breakfast, and so on, but no matter how good you feel, do not clean the house, vacuum, do laundry, pick up a heavy child, rearrange the attic, and so on! We do not want you to bleed and cause increased postsurgical swelling and bruising. This is the number-one cause of postsurgical problems. Many people do not take the limitation in activity seriously. They end up back in the operating room with a hematoma, with an infection, or an open incision. We have found that almost all complications occur in people who do not follow these rec- ommendations. There is no such thing in plastic surgery as a superhuman "good healer." How fast you recovered from a previous surgery does not apply to this procedure. You should have no events, dinners, ball games, child events, parties, trips to the mall, or travel planned for two weeks after surgery. No exceptions. Please realize that doing too* much too soon will set your healing back weeks or months, so it is simply not worth it.

*Ice packs:* Cold or ice packs help to reduce swelling, bruising, and pain. Use crushed ice and put the ice into a Ziploc bag, placed over a cloth. This should help, not hurt. If the ice feels too uncomfortable, don't use it as often.

*Diet:* If you have any postoperative nausea, carbonated sodas and dry crackers may settle the stomach. If nausea is severe, use the nausea medication that is in your medication kit, as directed on the bottle. If you feel normal, start with liquids and bland foods, and if those are well tolerated, progress to a regular diet. Remember that anesthesia paralyzes your stomach, so you will not digest quickly or feel hungry. This is okay. Listen to your body and do not force yourself. A good rule of thumb is to eat as if you have the flu—bland, easy-to-eat items only.

*Constipation:* Constipation is extremely common after surgery. It is due to the pain medication. This is why we would like you to change to Tylenol or acetaminophen as soon as possible. If symptoms persist for more than two days, use milk of magnesia or magnesium citrate, as directed on the bottle. These medications are available over the counter at all local stores. Milk of magnesia seems to work almost 95 percent of the time.

*Smoking:* Smoking reduces capillary flow in your skin. We advise you not to smoke at all during the first six weeks after surgery. Smoking will cause healing problems and necrosis of your skin. This is also true for second-hand smoke. If you *live with any smokers, make sure they do not smoke around you and do not come near you with nicotine on their clothes.*

*Alcohol: Alcohol dilates the blood vessels and could increase postoperative bleeding. Please do not drink any alcohol (beer, wine, etc.) until you have stopped taking the prescription pain medication, as the combination of pain medication and alcohol can be deadly. You should avoid all alcohol for the month after surgery.*

*Driving: Please don't drive for at least two days after general anesthesia or intravenous sedation or while taking prescription pain medication. Also, depending on what surgery you had, it may not be comfortable to drive. You should have full range of motion before you start driving.*

*Postoperative appointments: It is very important that you follow up at the office as directed after the surgery. We must see you within the first week of your procedure.*

## Long-Term Time Commitments

In addition to the time you'll need immediately after surgery to recover both physically and mentally, there are some long-term things you must consider to make sure you are realistic about the amount of time your recovery will take.

Focusing on your workout and diet routine is essential to having the best results after a body contouring procedure. All too often, people who have a tummy tuck or liposuction stay in recovery mode too long after their procedures and end up gaining weight. Sometimes, their ability to fit into a smaller dress size makes people think it's okay to have that morning doughnut or skip their workout.

Nothing could be further from the truth. Almost everyone has heard stories about people spending thousands of dollars on surgery only to gain all their weight back. You should be looking at plastic surgery as a *life* change, not just a body change. Exercise, weight loss, and healthy habits are all part of the life-changing experience that plastic surgery can be. Immediately after you are cleared by your surgeon (usually in four to six weeks), you need to get back to the gym and into a regular workout routine that includes strenuous physical exercise at least three times a week, combined with watching dietary habits and the weight on the scale.

The second long-term thing you want to think about is taking care of your scar. After the first month passes and you're feeling better, you'll still need time to pay attention to your scar so it heals properly. Depending on the procedure you've had and how invasive it was, you may be caring for your scar for up to a year (or longer) after your surgery. Many people don't realize incisions take a while to fade, and your scar care routine plays a huge factor in the final result you get. You should be asking your surgeon what he/she recommends and make the time and effort to be vigilant about your scar care. It will pay off in the long run.

Another important thing to plan for is the unexpected. You should think about what you will do if there is any sort of complication after your procedure that would add to your recovery time. Bleeding, infection, or healing problems can all add weeks to your recovery, for which you should have a contingency plan in place. Complications are rare in plastic surgery (if performed by an experienced professional), but they do happen, and they do lengthen your recovery period. Depending on what it is, a complication can add one to four weeks, or longer, to your recovery time. Complications also mean additional visits to your doctor, so you'll need time to get to the doctor, and you'll need someone to drive you there. You may need hospitalization or a caretaker at home. Have an honest conversation with your surgeon about what the plan would be for managing complications. Serious complications are rare, but you should always plan for the unexpected.

### Taking Care of Your Scar

Every time the skin is broken for any reason, traumatically or surgically, you *will always* get a scar. Your genetic healing ability has a lot to do with your healing, but you and your surgeon contribute to your final scar result. There is no such thing as no scar. The trick is to minimize the scar as much as possible by treating it aggressively *while* it is healing and to have the understanding that a scar can take a year or two to really fade. We tell all of our patients that no matter how well their surgery is done, there is always a chance of developing a scar. The trick is to do everything possible to *prevent it, treat it, and minimize it.*

### Preventing a Bad Scar

Many things can make a scar worse. Sometimes they can be avoided, and sometimes they cannot. For example, people with dark skin, hair, and eyes are prone to developing worse scars than people with lighter skin—and you can't change your genetic makeup. Also, certain medical conditions, such as diabetes, obesity, and scleroderma, can adversely affect scars. Smoking is one of the worst possible things you can do before and after a surgical procedure. If you smoke, chances are you will have a bad scar. Smoking has nicotine in it, which constricts blood vessels, and also carbon monoxide, which depletes your blood of the nourishment provided by oxygen. You should quit all nicotine products at least six weeks before your surgery or else all bets are off. Certain surgeries have a higher chance of healing problems than others. Any surgery where a flap of skin is developed (for example, a tummy tuck or a breast lift) needs extra special care to achieve good healing and minimal scarring. Overactivity immediately after a surgery is also bad for scars as it can pull on the scar and cause it to widen.

There are different problems a scar can have, and each problem is treated differently. It is very important to understand that there are different types of unsightly scars that require different kinds of prevention and treatment. For the purposes of an organized discussion, scars can be divided up into groups that include: thick scars, red scars, brown scars, white scars, wide scars, indented scars, and poorly hidden scars.

• *Thick scars:* Certain people are genetically prone to making "bad" scars. Believe it or not, these are actually people who are prone to overhealing. A scar is basically a collection of collagen, blood vessels, and epithelium (the outer layer of skin) trying to close a defect in the skin layer. Some individuals tend to lay down too much collagen, creating a thick red scar. This type of raised scar is called hypertrophic scarring. A keloid is an extreme type of hypertrophic scar that grows like a tumor beyond the borders of the original break in the skin.

We often find that many people mistake hypertrophic scars for keloids or even normal scars for keloids! Just because you think your scar could look better, doesn't mean it is a keloid. Hypertrophic and keloid scars do not always occur consistently. People prone to them can develop them after one surgery but not after the next surgery, or they can occur on certain parts of the body (the breast bone, joints, and scalp are especially prone) and not others. Hypertrophic scarring usually occurs in people who are genetically prone to it (African Americans, Asians, Italians, American Indians, Hispanics), basically almost all darker skin types. In fact, if you have blonde hair and blue eyes, you have a much better chance of your scar healing with no thickness to it at all. In general, the amount of collagen you have in your scar is at its greatest in six weeks to three months after the skin injury (or surgery), so this is the time to really make sure you do whatever you can to keep the scar flat. Irritation to your scar (from too much movement in the area or from tight clothing rubbing on the scar) can stimulate the scar to overheal and become hypertrophic.

*The treatment* involves pressure, silicone, and vitamin E. Constant pressure on the scar (either with tape or silicone gel sheeting) as well as massage in the first six months of healing can dramatically reduce the thickness of a scar. In general, we tell our patients to use a micropore tape for the first one to six months after surgery. Silicone gel sheets also help to accomplish the same goal. These products work especially well for people who are genetically prone to making hypertrophic or keloidal scars. Even old scars can be treated by pressure and massage, but remember it can take time. Finally, if all else fails and it has been over a year, consider laser resurfacing (using a laser to reduce the thick area) or scar revision (surgery to remove the scar, resuture it, and "try again!").

• *Red scars:* All scars are initially red. This is a totally normal phenomenon and is due to increased blood flow to the area and extra blood vessels forming to bring all the nutrients in your blood to the area that needs to heal. More blood flow means more redness, which is totally normal. In fact, the scar can, sometimes, take on a purplish hue. It is important to realize that even in the best of circumstances, redness only starts going away after seven months. It can take a year or longer for it to totally fade. People who have trouble with redness for a longer period of time are usually light complexioned and are the same people whose entire face turns a bright red when embarrassed or emotional. Vitamin E can decrease the amount of red in a scar. If you are in a hurry, you can get rid of redness more quickly with an IPL (intense pulsed light) treatment. Patience is usually the key, and with time it will get better.

**Dr. Shah Recommends**

voiding sun and tanning beds also helps to reduce the redness of a scar and prevents permanent discoloration of the scar.

• *Brown scars:* People with darker skin are also prone to produce more of the brown pigment called melanin, which is deposited preferentially around scars and causes what is known as hyperpigmentation of the scar. It can get worse with time and sun exposure. To minimize hyperpigmentation on a scar, a few things can work: you can use a prescription lightening cream such as hydroquinone, or you can peel the scar with products that contain onion extract or glycolic acid. It takes several months of this treatment to lighten a scar, which may never totally lighten to the same color of the surrounding skin.

• *White scars:* Usually, a thin white scar is the goal of any surgery. If the white really stands out (for example a scar around your areola), one option is to perform cosmetic tattooing of the scar. Scar camouflage is performed by matching the color of the surrounding skin with a tattoo done directly over the scar. It can take more than one treatment to adequately camouflage the scar, and it requires an artistic touch.

• *Wide scars:* Having thin skin, or just putting too much pull on a scar immediately after surgery (overactivity), can cause a wide scar. Plastic surgeons are especially good at preventing this from happening by using special suturing techniques to distribute the tension on the scar and provide it with the most support. The classic example of a widened scar is the stretch marks a woman may get after pregnancy. Any scar can become widened like a stretch mark. Too much tension on a scar after surgery (i.e., not resting!) during the critical first month of healing can lead to a scar widening. Use a special kind of tape to provide additional support to a scar during this first month. The tape helps to hold the scar together, and reminds you not to pull on it too much. If a scar still turns out to be wide, you can try an ablative laser (such as a $CO_2$ or an Erbium laser), or have it revised (redone) in surgery.

• *Indented scars:* A scar that indents catches light and creates a shadow in such a way that it becomes very noticeable. This usually occurs because there is additional scar tissue underneath the scar that is attaching it to deeper structures such as muscle or bone. In the initial stages of scar formation you can massage a scar to prevent it from attaching to these deep structures. However, if the scar has been indented for more than a year, you will need to have it surgically revised or filled with a dermal filler to make it better.

• *Poorly hidden scars:* Some scars, even though they have healed well, are just in a bad spot. Typical examples include the face or the décolleté. Sometimes, the only thing you can do is camouflage them with makeup (there are several brands of camouflage makeup that are specially designed to cover up scars) or employ some very special plastic surgery techniques (a Z-plasty is one example) to change the direction of, or to hide, these scars.

In summary, be healthy, follow these tips, and be patient with your healing process. Your scar will usually get better with time. You must give your scar at least one year to heal itself.

## Test Yourself

Make sure you can answer <u>yes</u> to all of these questions before you proceed.

1. Can I take enough time off work?

2. Can I take enough time away from parenting?

3. Can I put my life on hold and focus on recovery for the necessary amount of time?

4. Do my significant other, family members, and/or other care-takers have enough time to help me through my recovery?

5. Do I have a contingency plan in place should I experience a complication?

6. Am I committed to returning to the gym after I have totally healed?

7. Do I know what I need to do to take care of my scar after my surgery?

------------------------------

# Lack of a Support System

Having a plastic surgery procedure requires physical *and emotional* support. A support system built of understanding and able friends and family is a must following surgery. Ninety-eight percent of plastic surgery procedures are done in a "outpatient" setting, which means that you don't spend any time admitted into a hospital after your procedure. Once your pain is well controlled in the recovery room, and you are fully awake from the anesthesia, you will be "discharged" from the place where you had surgery. Your caretaker will be your family member or friend who has volunteered to take care of you.

To most, it makes sense to have help after surgery. However, some people mistakenly believe they'll be fine on their own. "I'm tough," "I heal fast," and "I don't need help" are a few comments I hear that I know can lead to a disaster. Let me give you a few reasons why you need help for at least two to three days after any surgical procedure.

First, let's discuss anemia and dehydration. After having anesthesia, as well as some blood loss and swelling, you will suffer some degree of dehydration (lack of water in your bloodstream) or anemia (a decreased number of red blood cells in your bloodstream). This combination of decreased blood count, decreased fluid volume, and residual anesthesia can lead to a high incidence   of fainting. In medicine, we refer to this as a "vaso-vagal episode" referring to the nerves involved in the response. As you know, when you faint, you lose complete control of your body and you fall. Many people can faint on stairs and tumble down, or faint in the bathroom and hit their head on the tub or sink. All of these situations can result in disastrous complications.  During the first three days after your surgery you want to make sure that every time you go to the bathroom or take a shower, someone is there in case you have a vaso-vagal episode.

Second, you should know that there's also a large amount of "brain fog" after any surgical procedure. You feel as though you can't think straight and you are easily forgetful. It truly helps to have someone else manage your medications and even help you keep time in perspective. You're going to be sleeping a lot. You  might wake up and not know if you took a pill five minutes earlier or six hours earlier. These situations can lead to underdosing or overdosing. You definitely want someone around to help with medication administration during these first few days while your brain stabilizes itself.

Different surgeries will cause various limitations. For example, if you have surgery of the face, you might not be able to see as well as you normally would due to swelling around your eyes. Someone might have to walk you to the bathroom or help you eat or drink because you literally can't see.

When you have upper body surgery, such as breast, arm, or abdominal surgery, you cannot get out of bed without help. People don't realize how much they use their chest and abdominal muscles for almost every daily task they do. That is why they are called your "core muscles." You want to be sure you have someone helping you get around the house after this kind of surgery since your core will be weak and prone to injury.

In addition to someone helping you recover, you will need someone to temporarily take over whatever personal responsibilities you have, both at work and around the house. You'll be stuck mostly in bed, which means you will need help for basic things such as meals, driving to the doctor, and chores around the house. If you want to recover properly and safely, you'll need to secure help and be comfortable with letting things go for a while. You have to remember that you do not have to vacuum, clean house, or cook a meal for a couple of weeks. Your family will survive on pizza, and your home will be just fine, despite the few crumbs on the floor.

## Planning Ahead

Another good idea is to make a list of your daily responsibilities and figure out who in the family is going to be taking them over well in advance of your surgery. Driving the kids to soccer games, making breakfast, and household chores are all things that someone else will have to take over for a while. It's often hard to remember what you do from day to day, so my advice is to keep a journal for a week of everything you do around the house and use this as a guideline for discussion at a family meeting. Create a list, and write their names next to their responsibilities. Who knows, you may even be able to get the kids to finally do the dishes!

One suggestion I make to all my patients is that, if possible, they should have a family member, such as a mother, aunt, or sister, come to help for a few weeks. That person should actually move in with the patient for a period of time because around-the-clock help will be required. Three to five days of consistant companionship will be needed after most surgical procedures. For some of the larger pro-cedures, such as a tummy tuck, patients will need someone available for a minimum of two weeks.

## Dr. Shah Recommends

You'll likely need constant help for three to five days after most surgical procedures. For some of the bigger procedures such as tummy tucks, you may need someone for as long as two weeks. If possible, have a helper move in with you for that period of time.

### Asking for Help

You should think long and hard about *whom* you ask to help you recover after your surgery. You may be able to ask your mother-in-law, for example, to help with the housework and kids, but that doesn't mean she is the right person to support you psychologically. The psychological support from all of your caretakers is extremely important in organizing your postoperative care plan.

Talking to your caretakers before surgery so they understand how to be encouraging and not negative is a must. Phrases like "I told you so" or "you did it to yourself" should never be uttered around the post-operative patient. For the first few weeks, when you look in the mirror after surgery, you're going to be swollen and bruised. Things are not going to look good in the beginning, but that's normal. You need someone who is going to remind you of that and be encourag-ing if you "freak out" about what you see, not someone who is going to make you feel worse.

Your caretakers should say, "Remember the doctor told you that you're going to be swollen. Don't worry right now. It will go away. Get some rest." If you don't have someone reminding you that, then you will start questioning yourself because you're in a vulnerable state. It is at this moment you need the most supportive person you know around you.

The person you choose should be readily available to assume the caretaker role starting the day of your surgery. He or she should accompany you to your surgery appointment and drive you home after surgery. This gives the caretaker the chance to talk to your surgeon and nurse to know exactly how to care for you and what to expect.

## Test Yourself

Make sure you can answer <u>yes</u> to all of these questions before you proceed.

1. Have you made a list of all the activities you'll need someone else to take care of following surgery?

2. Have you arranged for someone to take care of you full time (twenty-four hours a day) at least three to five days following surgery?

3. Do all the people helping you understand what their responsibilities will be?

4. Do all your caretakers understand how to be encouraging, and not negative, about the way you look and feel?

5. Have you arranged adequate transportation to and from the surgery center with someone you trust?

6. Do you have someone who can do all your household chores (laundry, cooking, vacuuming) for two to four weeks after your surgery? (Usually, all these chores are reassigned to family members.)

7. Have you arranged transportation to and from your postoperative visits to your surgeon?

8. Do you have a list of people who are readily available and whom you can call if you need help?

9. Do you feel comfortable telling at least one person at work (preferably your boss) that you are having a procedure and you may need additional time off if needed to ensure good recovery?

10. Did you explain to your trusted family, friends, and coworkers that, for the first six to twelve months after surgery, you would feel better if they do not comment negatively about your healing and results?

------------------------------

# Lack of Research

As you may have gathered from the last few chapters, undergoing plastic surgery is a big decision, not something to enter into lightly. And, just like any major decision in your life, you do not want to dive in without first doing your homework. That means not only knowing what's involved in the procedure and how to prepare for recovery but also doing some in-depth research on the surgeon you have chosen and the facility where the procedure will be done.

Hopefully, what you've read thus far, along with the quiz questions at the end of each chapter, has helped you with your research and preparation. Here are some additional tips that will help protect you when making the final big decision of your plastic surgery adventure, which concerns where your procedure will be done and who will do it.

## Recommendations

First, get recommendations from friends and family whom you trust. Recommendations are a great start, but remember that just because one person you talked to had one positive outcome doesn't mean that person did their research either. After noting your friends, reccommendations, search the Internet for reviews and other doctors in your area. Once you have made a list of doctors from your recommendations and online searches, you should make a short list of the ones that are your favorites and schedule a few consultations! Make sure you ask your prospective surgeons a few specific questions:

1. *"Have you done a fellowship in plastic and reconstructive surgery?"* This question will help you to weed out doctors who just did a weekend course in some procedure but don't have thorough formal training and experience in plastic surgery.

2. *"Are you board certified or board eligible for the American Board of Plastic Surgery?"* This will tell you if the doctor has undergone specific training in plastic surgery. This ensures that your surgeon has been properly trained according to the American Board of Medical Specialties.

3. *"How many of these procedures have you done?"* This question will give you an idea of the level of experience the doctor has in the specific procedure you are considering. For common procedures such as breast augmentation and tummy tucks you would expect a number in the hundreds. Doctors who have performed fewer procedures are not necessarily less competent. They may be new to the profession and therefore have not amassed a large number of procedures but are still technically competent.

4. *"Do you operate at an accredited surgery center or hospital?"* Make sure that your surgical procedure isn't being done in the back room of an office. To be performed under the safest possible condition, a plastic surgery operation must be done in a hospital or an accredited surgical facility. There are five organizations that certify facilities as safe for

conducting surgery: state certification, AAAHC, AAAASF, Medicare, and JCAHO. An operating room must have one of these certifications to meet the minimal criteria for surgery. Often, since there is no organization policing doctor offices, these procedures have been performed in an office environment that is not required to have the same safeguards as an accredited facility. Worse, there have been horror stories of procedures being performed out of a private home, spa, hair salon, or hotel room! This is simply not safe and should raise serious red flags.

5. *"Do you have privileges to do this procedure at a hospital?"* Hospitals have high standards and will do some of the vetting for you. If the hospital doesn't give a doctor privileges to do a procedure, it means that, for some reason, that doctor was deemed not properly trained or qualified to do the procedure.

A large regulatory gap we have in the United States is that it's not illegal for any doctor with an MD or DO degree to do any kind of procedure in the back room of his office. A gynecologist can do heart surgery in his office if he wanted to! It is not considered "illegal" until a medical board reprimands that physician for a complication or a complaint that occurred. A state medical board can take away a doctor's license to practice medicine after the fact (after someone complains, the board evaluates, and a long legal process results in a reprimand or the removal of the doctor's medical license). Often, this process takes years, and in the meantime, many doctors continue to practice cosmetic surgery they are not qualified to do. That puts the onus on the patient to do their research and not to assume that just because a procedure is advertised as being offered at a   particular physician's office, that they are qualified to do so. There are many examples in the media of the disastrous consequences of unquali-fied people performing surgery in uncertified facilities. Unfortu-nately, the law doesn't explicitly and proactively prevent that from happening. The only mechanisms in place that address these situa-tions are lawsuits and medical board actions, but, unfortunately, they take time. In the meantime, sadly, many people get hurt.

Reputable accredited surgical facilities require the doctors to whom they give privileges to have high standards. By ensuring your procedure will be performed at such a facility, you have additional evidence that your doctor has the right experience and qualifications.

## Surgery Facility

Research the facility where you are having the procedure. It's a good idea to ask how the facility handles emergencies in case something goes wrong. It's good to know whether the facility or hospital can handle a major emergency on-site or whether you'd need to be trans-ferred to another location. Most outpatient surgical facilities have policies and procedures in place for emergencies beyond their scope, and this often includes a transfer agreement to a nearby hospital.

## Fully Understanding Your Procedure
## and Postoperative Care

Make sure you have a full understanding of the procedure being performed and what sort of postoperative care you will need. The second half of this book will give you more specific information on the recovery associated with the most-common procedures. You should also ask your doctor to fully explain your postoperative care.

It's also a good idea to ask other people who have been through the procedure you're considering what it was like for them. Patients have a different perspective from that of doctors, so former patients are likely to tell you things the doctor wouldn't think of saying. In fact, I often suggest that if people know someone who's having a procedure done, they should volunteer to take care of that person so they can see firsthand what it's like. If you don't know someone who's had the procedure done, you can ask your doctor to put you in touch with former patients so you can ask questions. The Internet has many forums that also detail actual patient experiences.

## Realistic Expectations

Make sure you have realistic expectations for the results. Although this is discussed elsewhere in this book, it's worth repeating. Talking with former patients can help with this, but you should also research before and after photos. You can find many of these online and you can also ask your doctor to show you some as well. Many doctors will have pictures of people immediately after surgery, so you can see what's normal a few days after surgery. When looking at before and after pictures, try to find patients who looked like you before their surgery so you can realistically see what can be achieved for your body type.

## Preparation Checklist

Once someone has decided to go ahead with a procedure, we give that person the following checklist to help prepare. Read through it so you have a good idea of how to best prepare yourself. Remember, this is just a sample checklist for a specific procedure at our practice. Your surgeon may have a different set of instructions for your particular procedure. This checklist is simply provided as a guide to discussion between you and your surgeon. Overall, the key is to not rush into the decision to have surgery. Remember, you are permanently changing the way you look, but that doesn't mean that doing your research should feel overwhelming. Most patients can get all the information they need within a week if they're willing to invest the time and energy.

## PREPARING FOR SURGERY CHECKLIST

| START NOW | |
|---|---|
| | **STOP SMOKING:** You must completely stop smoking for a minimum of four to six weeks prior to surgery or your surgeon may decide not to perform surgery. Smoking *will cause* postoperative complications, including but not limited to: *thick scars, open wounds,* and *delayed healing.* |
| | **TAKE MULTIVITAMINS:** Start taking multivitamins daily to improve your general health once you have scheduled your surgery. Taking additional vitamin C is also helpful in promoting healing. |
| | **SEE YOUR PRIMARY CARE DOCTOR:** It is important that everyone involved in your health care knows of your decision to undergo surgery. Have a full physical performed as soon as possible. In certain situations (age over fifty, health issues, certain medications) you may require a cardiac evaluation, which should be completed *before* your pre-op visit. |
| | **DO NOT TAKE ASPIRIN OR IBUPROFEN:** Stop taking medications containing aspirin or ibuprofen for at least two weeks before surgery, and remain off them for at least two weeks after surgery.. These medications can cause bleeding problems during and after surgery. Instead, use medications containing acetaminophen (such as Tylenol). |
| YOUR PRE-OPERATIVE APPOINTMENT | |
| | **THINGS TO BRING:** Bring a list of all of the medications you are taking (vitamins, herbals, prescriptions, over-the-counter). |
| | Plan to spend at least one hour listening carefully to the instructions. Bring your caretaker with you to this appointment. |
| ONE TO TWO WEEKS BEFORE SURGERY | |
| | **ORDER YOUR GARMENT:** With some procedures you will need to purchase a garment. Make sure you place this order ASAP as it sometimes takes a week or longer to receive the garment. |

| | |
|---|---|
| | **GET YOUR TRANSPORTATION ARRANGED:** You must be discharged from the facility to the care of an adult family member or friend after your surgery. You cannot drive yourself home. It is important to have a car that is easy to get in and out of after your surgery. |
| | **GET YOUR ERRANDS, CHILD CARE, AND HOUSEHOLD AFFAIRS ARRANGED:** Plan on not being able to do much for two weeks after surgery. Make sure someone will be responsible for cleaning, child care, driving you around, and so on, after surgery. |
| | **NOTIFY YOUR WORKPLACE:** Notify your workplace of how much time you need off, but let them know you may require additional time if your doctor recommends it. |
| | **COMFORT ITEMS:** Consider buying or renting a walker, ice packs, wedge pillow, a small bell, and other items you can think of to make your recovery more comfortable. Buy books and movies you've been wanting to catch up on because you'll be physically inactive for a while. |
| | **BUY BROMELAIN AND ARNICA:** Arnica montana and bromelain (a natural ingredient found in pineapples) are available at most pharmacies and health food stores. They help to reduce swelling and bruising. Start to take them before your surgery. |
| | **BUY CONTRACEPTIVES:** Antibiotics can make oral birth control pills less effective. You may want to buy additional forms of contraception to use during the month or two after surgery. Barrier methods such as condoms are recommended. |
| **DAY BEFORE SURGERY** | |
| | **BUY ANTIBACTERIAL SOAP:** It is important to take a shower with antibacterial soap (Dial, for example) the day before surgery. If you are having abdominal surgery, clean your belly button thoroughly with antibacterial soap and a Q-tip. |
| | **TAKE YOUR MEDICATIONS:** You should have already started the arnica and bromelain two days before surgery. (This may be completely different for your doctor.) |
| | **DO NOT EAT OR DRINK AFTER MIDNIGHT:** Do not take any food or drink by mouth (including water) after midnight on the night before surgery. |
| | **REMOVE ALL BODY PIERCINGS:** Remove all body piercings *prior to the day of surgery.* If you arrive at the surgery center with body jewelry of any type, metal or otherwise, you will be sent home and your surgery may be cancelled. |

| | |
|---|---|
| | **REMOVE ACRYLIC NAILS AND ALL JEWELRY:** This is very important. Acrylic nails have been shown to dramatically increase infection rate and jewelry is not allowed to be worn in surgery. Leave all jewelry at home, including your wedding ring. |
| | **CONFIRM YOUR TRANSPORTATION:** Be absolutely sure your transportation driver is an adult over the age of eighteen who can be with you the entire time before and after surgery. Only one person should come with you to the center. |
| | **CONFIRM YOUR CARETAKER:** Be absolutely sure your caretaker is available to stay with you for at least twenty-four to forty-eight hours after surgery. |
| | **GET SOME SLEEP:** Make sure to plan to get a good night's sleep before surgery. |
| **MORNING OF SURGERY** | |
| | **SHOWER:** You should shower the night before surgery and again on the morning of surgery, with antibacterial soap. You may brush your teeth, but do not swallow the water. Do not use any *lotion, underarm deodorant, makeup,* or *hair products.* |
| | **ATTIRE:** The only acceptable attire is loose-fitting pajamas that button in the front, socks, and slip-on shoes or slippers. Please come to the surgery center wearing them and a robe if you like. |

**Test Yourself**

Make sure you can answer <u>yes</u> to all of these questions before you proceed.

1. Have I checked out my physician, and do I have confidence in his experience and abilities?

2. Have I checked out the facility where the procedure will be performed, and do I know whether it's a reputable, accredited hospital or surgical center?

3. Do I have a full understanding of the procedure I will undergo?

4. Do I have a full understanding of what the recovery process will be like?

5. Do I have realistic expectations of the results?

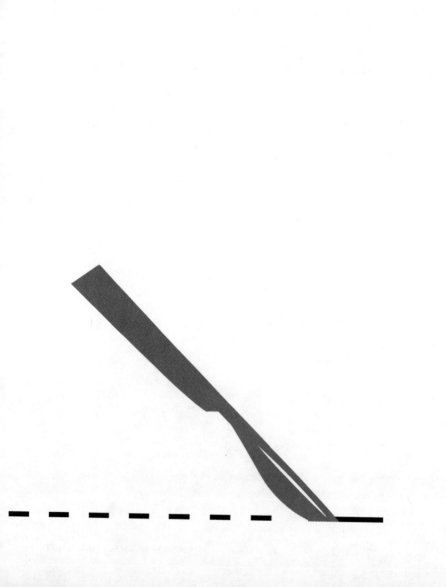

# PART 2

-------------------------

# What You Should Know before Going Forward

I f you have read through part 1 of this book and answered all the quiz questions at the end of each chapter, you can feel good about moving forward. Part 2 will give you more specific information about the procedure you're considering so that you can further your research and set yourself up for success.

------------------------------------

# CHAPTER 1

# Facial Procedures

Facial surgery is done to smooth wrinkles, lift sagging skin on various areas of the face, or remove excess skin around the eyes or in other places. There are many different procedures that are in a plastic surgeon's tool box that can affect specific areas of concern. One major misconception that many patients have is that a face lift is going to affect your entire face from the brow to the chin. In reality, a full facial rejuvenation often includes a range of different procedures in combination, with the face lift only being one of those procedures. These procedures are:

1. *A brow lift:* a lift and sometimes removal of the skin covering the area above your eyebrows to the top of your forehead.

2. *An eyelid lift:* a removal of loose skin covering your upper and lower eyelids, with occasionally some manipulation of the fat underneath.

3. *A face lift:* a tucking and removing of the skin covering mainly your cheek and jowl areas.

4. *A neck lift:* a tucking and removing of the skin covering your neck area. (This procedure is rarely done separately

from a face lift, a "neck lift" is basically an extension of the face lift procedure into the neck area.)

5.  *A fat transfer:* moving fat from one area of your body into the face to replace fat that has dissipated with time.

Each one of these is a separate procedure, so a specific discussion with your doctor about your expectations and what areas are bothering you is essential. A face lift won't change your brow or your neck (although many surgeons will perform a neck lift with every face lift). A brow lift doesn't mean the doctor will work on that extra skin that some people get on their upper eyelids or on the bags beneath the eye. People often get confused about the terminology involved, so it is important to be specific about exactly what is bothering you by pointing to the areas in a mirror while you and your surgeon are discussing these various areas of concern.

The various facial procedures can be done individually or you can have multiple procedures done at the same time. If you want to target more than one area, or the entire face, it's better to do them together because then you only go through one recovery period and one anesthetic. On the other hand, some people have only one very specific problem area they want to fix, so focusing only on that area is the right thing to do.

As you can imagine, the face is the most complex area of cosmetic plastic surgery and requires a surgeon who has extensive experience in facial procedures. There are key specialties that focus on the face, and you should do your research to be sure to choose a properly trained provider. These specialties include the following:

•   board-certified plastic surgeons
•   board-certified facial plastic surgeons (a subspecialty of ear, nose, and throat surgeons)

- board-certified oculoplastic surgeons (a subspecialty of physician ophthalmologists)

Note that all three of these specialists are physicians (MD or DO) and have board certifications approved by the American Federation of Medical Boards.

## The Procedures

### BROW LIFT

A brow lift focuses on the area above your upper eyelids. This includes some very specific areas of concern: the eyebrows (and the descent of this area), the horizontal wrinkles above the brow, the vertical wrinkles between the brows (also known as glabella lines), the hairline, and the amount of skin (or space) of the brow.

Most people seek help for this area of the face when they feel they look "tired" or "angry." Usually looking "tired" involves descent of the brow. You can tell your brow has descended, a normal occurrence of aging, by the location of your eyebrow hair in relationship to the bony prominence there (the supraorbital rim). For men, the eyebrow should be right on top of this orbital rim. Women usually like to have their eyebrow above the rim. If your brow has descended below this level, you may require a brow lift.

Many people reflexively raise their brow with their brow muscle when their brow begins to descend and obstruct their vision. This can cause vertical lines to appear in the brow that create a more aged look.

In general, there are two different ways of doing a brow lift: the open method and the endoscopic method. The open method involves making an incision in (or just at) your hairline, trimming the excess skin, and stitching the two sections back together. The endoscopic method involves lifting the brow through two small incisions in your hairline, using a camera to "release" your brow, and then putting some sort of anchor underneath the skin—either a suture anchor tied to a tiny screw or an absorbable synthetic anchor—to hold the brow up. Your doctor will help you choose which method will work best for you, but generally, if your brow has a lot of extra skin that should be removed, you are likely to need the "open" method.

During your discussion of this procedure with your surgeon, you should find out the answers to these questions:

1.  Which procedure (open or endoscopic) would be the best method for me?
2.   Will I need to have any skin removed?
3.  What will be done about the vertical lines and glabella lines?
4.  Will I be able to move my brow after the surgery?
5.  What will happen to my hairline?
6.  What will be the shape of my eyebrows afterward?
7.  What are potential complications of this procedure, and what are the treatment options for those complications?
8.  Would I be able to get a similar result with Botox™ or any other non-invasive procedure?

In general, a brow lift is a relatively straightforward procedure if performed by an experienced surgeon with proper training. Complications are rare, and a brow lift can take years off your appearance.

## EYELID LIFTS

One of the most talked-about areas in any beauty magazine is the eyes. The eyes (or the skin and tissue around the eyes) often display the first signs of aging as we grow older. As such, much of plastic surgery literature is devoted to the rejuvenation of this delicate but beautiful part of the face. The eyelids include both the upper and the lower eyelids. Believe it or not, this relatively small area of our bodies has intricate anatomical details that require precise adjustments, often as small as one millimeter!

As people age, they sometimes get extra skin on their upper eyelids that can look loose and crepey. With an upper eyelid lift, we're not actually lifting anything. The procedure involves removing this excess skin (sometimes only 1–2 mm of skin), possibly removing fat, occasionally adjusting the position of the tear gland, and sometimes adjusting the attachment points of the eyelid to the deeper structures. An upper eyelid lift is done first by making an incision in the crease of your eyelid, followed by the delicate procedures described above and then suturing the skin together.

The same adjustments can also be made with extra skin and "bags" that form underneath the eyes in the lower eyelid area. A lower eyelid lift is done through an incision made right underneath the lid if the doctor is removing loose skin. If the doctor is only removing extra fat that's causing bags, he/she can actually hide the incision on the inside of the eyelid, where it will be invisible.

As you can imagine, eyelid lifts can be extremely complex procedures if someone is not intimately familiar with the anatomy. Thankfully, much of a plastic surgeon's training is focused on this area. When discussing surgery of this area, you must discuss all of the following:

1. Will skin be removed? If so where?
2. Where will the incisions be? Will they be visible?
3. Besides skin removal, what else will be done?
4. What about the wrinkles on the side of my eye (crow's feet)?
5. If fat is to be removed, will I get a "hollowed out" look to my eyes?

6. What are the possible complications of this procedure, and how are they handled?
7. How long will I be black and blue?
8. How long before I can read or drive?

## FACE LIFT

One of the most talked about procedures in the media, at hair salons, and even among plastic surgeons is the face lift. This procedure is also one of the least understood by the general public due to misrepresentation in the media.

What is a "face lift?" Although many think that the procedure is an overall rejuvenation of the entire face, the actual plastic surgery definition is a rejuvenation of the cheek and jowl areas of the face. To perform a face lift, an incision is made in front of your ear and extends underneath your earlobe toward the back of your scalp. The surgeon can then remove a small amount of loose skin, pull the skin tighter and occasionally tighten the underlying structures, and finally, suture the skin back together around the ear.

When people think of a face lift, they often think of the overtightened faces of celebrities. The reality is that most people who have had a face lift have a natural, rejuvenated look. Since a few millimeters can make the difference between a tightly pulled look and a natural look, it is important that you discuss your desires with your surgeon.

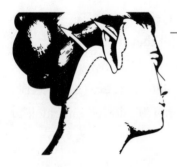

## NECK LIFT

A neck lift is rarely performed unless combined with a face lift. Some people look at their neck and think that they only "need" a neck lift. However, this is rarely the case. The skin of the face and neck act as a unit (meaning one cannot be moved without the other being moved), and tightening one without the other can lead to a mismatch in outcomes. A neck-lift incision goes into the hairline at the back of your head up to the base of ear. The doctor then pulls up the skin on the neck to smooth the jaw line and below. Occasionally, a separate incision is made under the chin to tighten the muscles and remove fat in that area. The platysma muscle is tightened via this incision because it has separated and caused bands under your neck.

## Length of Procedures

Eyelid lifts and brow lifts generally take one to two hours. Face lifts, neck lifts, or combinations of these procedures can last anywhere from three to eight hours.

## Realistic Expectations

- "Lifting" surgery procedures will only take care of saggy skin and help with wrinkles, but they're not going to take care of skin discoloration issues. If you have problems with the quality of your skin—sun damage, color splotches, melisma, acne scars, and so on—you should be talking to your doctor about the possibility of having a laser procedure, a chemical peel, or another type of skin resurfacing procedure in combination with your face lift. (See chapter 7 for more on this topic.) The quality of your skin is an important factor in the assessment of the results of any facial surgery and should be a major point of consideration when you are planning a facial surgery.

- When some people think of face lifts, they often think of Hollywood celebrities such as Joan Rivers or Kenny Rogers, but those celebrities' face lifts are not typical. Overtightening is often the result of multiple procedures, which causes scar tissue and problems with healing. Sometimes, people request a very dramatic result. You must have a conversation with the doctor about how you want your results to look because if you do want to look pulled, which some people do, you should communicate this to your doctor. If you want to look very natural, you should say that too because the amount of skin that's removed and the amount of pulling that is done in the operating room is under the doctor's control.

- Sometimes, people overestimate how much a face lift can turn back the clock. We may be able to move the clock back as much as twenty years, but trying to turn it back forty years is unrealistic. Facial aging is due to a combination of factors. Skin quality, volume loss, wrinkling, and sagging all play a part. Not all of these can be addressed simultaneously and completely. In addition, it simply is not possible to be seventy years of age and expect to look twenty. If someone promises you an extreme result, you should ask more questions.

- A face lift won't stop the aging process or prevent gravity from working on you. Eventually, the skin will settle, and gravity will continue its work in causing sagging and volume loss. You can slow down the effects of aging with a face lift, but you're still going to see changes over time. Some people even come back and have their face lifts redone after ten to twenty years.

- The effects of a face lift will last longer on some people than on others. It really depends on the elasticity of your skin. If, in a couple years, you feel that things have loosened up, that's not because the procedure was incorrectly done; it may be because your skin elasticity is not that great. There are some skin tightening lasers out there that can be effective for poor skin elasticity (see chapter 7 for more information), and taking care of your skin and staying out of the sun helps too, but a lot depends on your genes.

- Don't think your mini face lift will mean a faster recovery. A lot of people think adding the word *mini* to *surgery* means it's "hardly surgery at all." Nothing could be further from the truth. A mini face lift can help someone who doesn't have much skin to remove and doesn't need much neck tightening, but it's still a surgical face lift. Even though the scar might be a little bit shorter, it's almost exactly the same procedure as doing a regular face lift, and the recovery time is about the same.

- Some television ads promote branded face lifts that claim to make you look better and get you back to normal life within a day. Beware of those ads because that claim is totally unrealistic. Having a face lift is a major life experience, and it's going to take a month out of your life to fully recover to the point that you feel that you can go about your normal everyday tasks. Don't try to fit the procedure into a long weekend. It takes six to twelve months to see the final results of a face lift.

- Plastic surgery is a field associated with many new procedures and, frequently, hype about the "latest thing." Often, these procedures are just fads, and you'll end up paying a lot for little reward. Sometimes, they can even be dangerous. You can avoid a lot of problems by making sure you go to a reputable, board-certified plastic surgeon. Also, wait a little while (about a year) to allow newly advertised procedures to "flush" themselves out. The Internet will be full of reviews a year after you start hearing about a new procedure, and these can be useful in guiding your decision. Never assume that just because a procedure is marketed on television and the radio, it is safe or efficacious. Unfortunately, the law has not caught up with cosmetic surgery marketing, and many unsafe and ineffective procedures are promoted heavily.

- Lifting procedures won't help certain areas of your face. Wrinkles around your mouth (sometimes referred to as smokers' lines) are not treated with a face lift. The deep fold between your nose and mouth, called the nasolabial fold, may persist after your surgery. Deeply engrained wrinkles in the chin, between the brows, and in the forehead will also continue to be present after your face lift.

## How to Prepare Physically

- We prepare our patients' skin by putting them on a medical-grade skin care regimen prior to any of these facial procedures.

- You absolutely must stop smoking a month before the procedure. Be prepared to stay off cigarettes for at least a month after, hopefully forever.

- You must stay off any blood-thinning medications such as aspirins or ibuprofen for a month before and after the surgery.

- You want to stay out of the sun and out of sun-tanning booths for a month before and at least six months after the surgery.

- It's very important to prepare to take time off work. The length of time depends on how much you want to hide from others the fact that you've had a procedure done, but plan on taking at least two to four weeks after such a procedure and longer if you want to make sure all the telltale signs are gone before you show your face. It can take four weeks or longer before some people feel comfortable going out in public.

- You need to be aware that it can take six months to a year before the swelling goes away completely.

- Some people get very concerned about numbness in their face after surgery. You have to keep telling yourself that it's normal and will eventually go away.

### How to Prepare Mentally

- Have a really good conversation with your surgeon about where the scars are going to be placed and how visible they will be. You don't want to be surprised by your scar and how visible it is.

- It's important to understand that you'll likely feel nervous about going out in public after the surgery. In reality, people won't be able to see a big difference after two to four weeks even though you may feel they can because your face still feels numb and swollen. Actually, it never looks as bad as you think it does.

- You want to make sure that the people around you know that you're going to look different afterward (e.g., family and close coworkers), especially if you've had major procedures done. It's good to have a conversation beforehand to prepare them for that.

- You want to have an honest conversation with your loved ones about how looking different and looking younger will affect your relationship. Some people are resistant to it because they don't want their spouse to look younger than they do. Have that honest conversation before the surgery, and make sure there are no ill feelings that could lead to your significant other being resentful and not as supportive as he/she needs to be.

- After the surgery, you will be bruised and swollen, which will be tough to look at. Kids, especially, should be warned, or they should go somewhere else for the first few days. The bruising and swelling could scare children and other caretakers. It is important to see pictures of what it will look like afterward so everyone is prepared.

### Recovery and Results

Recovery time will be pretty much the same whether you're doing one procedure or many (which is why the majority of people elect to do multiple facial procedures at the same time). For at least two to three days, you're going to need help to move around the house because the swelling can make it hard to see, particularly with eye procedures.

All your rituals for cleaning and caring for your facial skin and putting on makeup are going to go out the window for a couple of weeks. You want to really baby your face and minimize how much you touch it during that time.

There are some special brands of makeup you can use a few days after surgery to cover up some of the bruising, but there's nothing that's going to make you look normal a few days afterward. Do not try to overapply makeup to cover the bruising, as this can lead to infections and other issues.

Some doctors will use a drain placed under the skin of your face at the time of surgery, especially if you have had a neck lift. A drain is a tube that comes out of the back of your incision to pull excess fluid and blood away from the facial flaps. The drain is usually removed a few days after your surgery. Not all doctors use it, but depending on the extent of your surgery, you might need one.

The scars from these procedures are usually well hidden after a few weeks. There are stitches that usually come out a few days after your surgery. It is important to give scars a year or longer to achieve maximal fading.

For most eyelid surgery, you're not going to be able to wear contact lenses for at least a week. You'll probably want to put some cooling packs on your eyes for a couple of days. Have your glasses available for the first few days after surgery. It is very important to rest your eyes after any eye surgery. It will be uncomfortable to read books and watch television. You're going to need to do more sleeping than anything else. Listening to the radio or books-on-tape is a good alternative.

## Possible Complications

Facelift surgery has some specific risks in addition to the *general* risks already described in previous chapters.

- *Numbness:* When the skin is separated from the underlying tissues during surgery, small sensory nerves are cut. Varying degrees of numbness will be present after surgery and will improve gradually as the nerves reconnect to the skin. This process can take two months for the face, neck, and cheeks, and nine to twelve months for the

### Personal Experience

I once saw a famous male celebrity patient who had had a face lift done with great, dramatic results. But he was upset that he wasn't featured in magazines afterward as his similarly aged contemporary Kenny Rogers had been after his face lift. Our surgeon refused to operate on him to pull his facial skin tighter. All explanations of the risks of over-pulling fell on deaf ears. The patient then went to another surgeon and had another face lift done. Unfortunately, he was pulled too tight and ended up having skin loss of about 5 mm on one side of his face. Although he eventually healed, the interim six months were awful for him.

One of the tenants of plastic surgery is "the enemy of good is better." This means that if it looks good, don't try to go for more, because you could risk complications and problems every time you go under the knife.

forehead and scalp. Some areas may remain numb for a longer time.

- *Tightness:* Frequently, there is a tight feeling in the neck, after a face lift. During surgery, not only the skin but also the underlying muscles are tightened to create a better and longer-lasting result. Additionally, the swelling will move downward in the first week and the neck will feel even tighter. Do not be alarmed! You will not choke, and the sensation will decrease during the first month.

- *Healing of sensory nerves:* As the nerves regenerate, itching, burning, tingling, and shooting sensations will occur. Ice, moisturizers, and gentle massaging are helpful during this phase of the healing process.

- *Firmness under skin:* Some degree of firmness or lumpiness under the skin is normal after surgery and will resolve with time. Local massage will speed resolution of this problem, which normally takes two to six months to disappear completely.

- *Asymmetric swelling:* Do not be alarmed if one side of your face is slightly more swollen or numb than the other. This is common and usually disappears within a few weeks.

- *Eye symptoms:* Even if they have not been operated on, your eyelids may feel tight because of the swelling that occurs in the entire face. Your vision may also be blurred from the ointment that is placed in them for protection during surgery. Eye drops and ice packs will feel particularly soothing for the first few days after surgery.

- *Activities:* Most patients who have had face lifts feel reasonably normal within three to four days after surgery even though they are swollen. If you wish to do light office work, you may. Do not, however, do any heavy activities or aerobic exercise for at least four weeks after surgery! Strenuous activities can cause bleeding and swelling for a longer period than is necessary.

- *Incisions (scars):* In the temple area, your doctor can make the incisions within the hairline or in front of the hairline. If made in front, the scars will be visible but the hairline will not change. Scars made within the hairline cause the hair to move up and slightly backward when the lift is done. We find it best to place the preauricular (in front of the ear) scar behind the tragus (the small flap at the external opening of the ear), as that incision is least noticeable. The incision behind the ear can also be made within or below the hairline. If made within the hairline, much of the scar will be hidden, *but there will be a change in the hairline and there will be more hair-free skin behind your ear.* If your doctor places the incision below the hairline, the hairline will remain intact, but the scar will be visible if you wear your hair up. Longer, rather than shorter, facelift incisions can produce a better result as more skin can be removed. On the other hand, longer incisions and more skin removal mean that more changes will occur in the hairline if the incisions are placed there. Your surgeon can attempt to reapproximate the hairline behind the ear and eliminate the notching but usually at the expense of the overall facelift result.

- *Hematoma:* If excessive bleeding occurs under the skin after surgery, a collection of blood under the skin (a hematoma) can form. This can be especially common if you have high blood pressure or vomit or cough excessively after surgery. If the hematoma remains small, the body will absorb it gradually. If it becomes larger, it may need to be removed by suction in the operating room. Further surgery to remove clots is uncommon but, occasionally, necessary.

- *Loss of sensation:* Permanent numbness rarely occurs. When it does, it usually involves the earlobes and rarely the skin in front of the ears.

- *Skin loss:* Occasionally, poor circulation coupled with skin under tension will lead to blistering, redness, and, rarely, small areas of skin loss. Skin loss most commonly occurs behind the ears but can occur elsewhere. If this happens, it will delay healing, and superficial scarring may occur. You may require some "touch-up" procedures. (This is why we ask smokers to discontinue smoking for several weeks before and after surgery, as they are at the greatest risk for this complication).

- *Postoperative sagging:* Your surgeon will walk a tightrope during surgery. If the skin is pulled too tight, circulation diminishes and skin can die. Your surgeon will lift or tighten your skin as much as it is safe to do. If your skin does not have normal elasticity, it may stretch or sag sooner than desired. This is not your surgeon's fault. A subsequent small tuck can be very helpful if you have this kind of skin.

- *Nerve injury:* It is extremely rare for the main trunk of the facial nerve to be injured. Temporary damage to one of the peripheral branches is uncommon. If this should happen, you might have difficulty in moving your forehead, upper lip, or lower lip. Resolution usually occurs in a month or two. However, permanent damage remains a remote possibility. Occasionally, the sensory nerve that supplies the earlobe may incur damage despite the best efforts to preserve its function.

- *Asymmetry:* No one's face is totally symmetrical. Many people notice asymmetry for the first time when they scrutinize themselves after a face lift. Because this surgery is as much an art as a science, surgical asymmetries can occur. Further surgery is rarely necessary.

- *Chronic pain:* Most facelift procedures cause very little discomfort for more than a few days, and all the skin sensation will have returned to normal in three to five months. In very rare cases, patients have noted chronic pain at the surgical site that lasts a year or longer (occasionally longer). Rarely, patients complain that the operated areas become superficially hot or red. These symptoms can occur following exercise or for no apparent reason and can occur over several months. The reasons for all the above symptoms are unclear and specific treatment is not known. Massage and ice packs may be symptomatically helpful. Some patience and understanding while the symptoms clear over time is required.

- *Swelling and pain in the parotid area:* The surface of the parotid gland (a large salivary gland below and in front of the ear) is exposed as part of the procedure for tightening the deeper layers. Occasional swelling of the parotid gland or discomfort while eating may occur for one to four weeks after surgery. This is a self-limiting problem and will resolve without treatment.

- *Scars:* Scars will occur and may go from pink and firm to faded and soft over a period of six to twelve months; some scars may widen, become depressed, or appear raised, firm, and "ropey" red, which may take two years or longer to fade and soften; scars will be permanent and visible.

- *Hair loss:* Some hair loss along the incisions lines on the scalp is possible.

- *Fluid collections:* Fluid collections may accumulate under the skin and may require drainage or aspiration (withdrawal by needle).

- *Injury to deeper structures:* Blood vessels, nerves, and muscles may be injured during a facelift procedure. The incidence of such injuries is rare (see "nerve injury" above).

- *Alternatives:* The face lift is an elective procedure, so not doing anything is a viable alternative. Chemical peels, laser resurfacing, and liposuction procedures may provide some degree of benefit but have their own risks. Noninvasive skin tightening treatments are also available. All of these are good options in some situations. Make sure you understand your options and why the face lift may or may not be the best operation for you.

## BEFORE AND AFTER

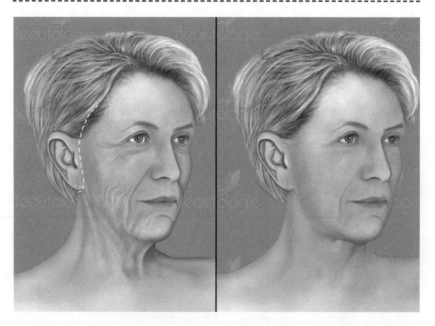

-------------------------------

# CHAPTER 2

# Rhinoplasty

Not all nose jobs are the same. When you have rhinoplasty surgery, or what's commonly called a nose job, there are many different aspects of your nose your doctor can work on. The surgeon can change the width of your nose, reduce the hump of the nose, and fix a crooked nose, and finally, there's the tip of the nose. The surgery can be customized depending on what results are sought, so it's important to have a clear conversation with your doctor about what you're looking for and what can realistically be achieved. It's helpful to bring pictures of noses that you like, but you should keep in mind that a nose that looks good on someone else won't necessarily fit your face. An in-depth conversation about the specific maneuvers that the surgeon will use and what can be accomplished is essential at your consultation.

## The Procedure

There are two different methods of performing a rhinoplasty procedure: open and closed. Open rhinoplasty exposes the nasal bone and cartilage structure of the nose by peeling back the skin of the nose. Closed rhinoplasty is done more by a surgeon's feel, and the skin is not removed from the cartilage and bones. Rather, a small incision is made inside your nostrils, and modifications are made through this incision. Whether you have an open or closed procedure depends on the extent of the surgery you need to make the changes you want. If you want extensive changes, your doctor will probably do an open rhinoplasty. However, if you just want a little work done on the tip, you will probably have a closed rhinoplasty.

The incisions for a rhinoplasty are generally well hidden at the bottom of your nose and inside your nostrils.

## Length of Procedure

Depending on the complexity of your surgery, a rhinoplasty can be performed in two to four hours, although it sometimes takes longer.

## Realistic Expectations

- It is very important to realize that your nose must be suited to your face. The overall shape and dimensions of your face, your ethnicity, your skin type, and many other factors determine the shape and size of nose that would "fit" your face. This is why there are hundreds of different kinds of noses. Angelina Jolie may have a nice nose, but it wouldn't work on Oprah Winfrey's face.

- Another important fact to accept is that only so much can be done to change the shape and size of your nose. It is almost impossible to give you exactly the nose you see on someone else. What your final result turns out to be has a lot to do with what the surgeon has to work with.

- It can be hard for patients to get a good picture of what the results will be, so doctors sometimes use computer programs to simulate the outcome. It's important to understand that these programs will not give you an exact image of what your nose will look like. In reality, a person's tissues, cartilages, and bones can react in unanticipated ways to a surgeon's work. Do not think of the computer simulation as a guarantee. More likely than not, after the surgery, your nose will look different from the computer simulation.

- Many people are extremely picky about their nose because it's right there in the center of their face, and they can spend a lot of time looking at it and feeling it. You have to keep in mind that what you are feeling and seeing is *your* perception. Others will not see the minor imperfections you see. You'll probably be more critical about the results than other people will be. Maybe, one side feels a little bit different than the other or there's a slight asymmetry, but those sorts of things are normal and to be expected.

- In the case of rhinoplasty, patience is extremely important. It really does take a year to see the final results, and any judgment of the final outcome before that year is over is unrealistic

## How to Prepare Mentally and Physically

- If you have any kind of psychological disorder or suspect you might have one, such as obsessive-compulsive disorder or bipolar disease, you want to make sure you've spoken to a psychologist to ensure this problem is under control before having the procedure. That's true of any plastic surgery but particularly true of rhinoplasty because people can often become fixated on their noses. If you are overly concerned about minor imperfections on your face, you really should have a talk with a psychiatrist to assess if you are ready for a rhinoplasty.

- You need to be mentally prepared for the fact that this surgery can have a long recovery period. Swelling on the nose takes a particularly long time to go away. As mentioned above, it's often as long as a year before you can see the final outcome. That means patience is the key to this procedure.

- Rhinoplasty is more obvious than other types of plastic surgery. People are going to notice you look different. You'll want to talk to them beforehand so that the change is not a surprise. That means talking not just to your immediate family but to all of your friends and work colleagues too because they'll probably also notice the difference in you.

- You want to tell the people who are close to you not to be judgmental for the first six months to a year. Things will continue to remodel and change during that period, so you and those around you need to let everything settle before you get a good picture of what you will look like. If people are judgmental about how you look, you're going to be much more sensitive about it.

### Recovery and Results

Rhinoplasty can be relatively simple if you're just having the closed procedure for a bit of work on the tip of your nose, or it can be a rather large surgery if bone resetting or major reshaping of the bulk of your nose is involved. Because of that, there's a range in terms of what you can expect for the cost of the procedure, the amount of time it takes to do, and of course, recovery. In general, the more you have done, the longer you're going to be recovering.

For a closed rhinoplasty, the recovery period can be as short as a week or two. For an open rhinoplasty with lots of changes to the nose, recovery can take two to four weeks.

If you have incisions inside the nose during an open procedure, for the first week you may have a hard time breathing and blowing your nose. You may feel very stuffy for the first week. Your doctor may even use nasal packing (gauze inside your nose) for a few days after the surgery.

### Risks

- *Internal scarring:* Internal scarring or adhesions may occur but are not a common complication.

- *Numbness:* Numbness will usually occur at the tip of your nose and will gradually decrease when the swelling decreases. The numbness usually gets better with time but not always.

- *Nasal obstruction:* Healing problems may cause a blockage to the airway, obstructing the nasal passage and causing difficulty in breathing.

- *Injury to adjacent structures and nasal function:* Injury to adjacent nerves, muscles, tear ducts, or blood vessels is rare. Alterations to your sense of smell can occur but are rare.

- *Perforated nasal septum:* A permanent hole (aka perforation) to the nasal septum (the firm area between your nostrils) is a rare complication. The perforation can be small and asymptomatic or large and require surgical correction.

- *Voice changes:* Changes in your voice may occur but are very rare.

- *Difficulty breathing through your nose:* Swelling will occur on the inside and outside of your nose. If surgery is also performed on your septum, you may have plastic splints sutured to the inside of your nose. The swelling and the splints will make it difficult to breathe through your nose. You will also have dried blood and debris inside your nostrils that will make it difficult to breathe through your nose.

- *Need for further surgery:* If asymmetry or an undesired contour is present, there may be a need for further surgery. There is no way to predict how the nose will heal over time. If a second procedure is necessary, it should be performed at least six months after the last nasal surgery, preferably a year to allow all the swelling to go away.

## Real-World Experience

Many people recall Michael Jackson when they think about rhinoplasty. His story is a perfect example of one of the tenets of plastic surgery: once something is good enough, you want to leave it alone. The body does not like having surgery in the same area multiple times. When a rhinoplasty is performed, blood vessels are cut, and you rely on other blood vessels to take over and supply the tissues with blood. If you do a surgery over and over again and keep cutting those blood vessels that are filling in for the other blood vessels, pretty soon you have no blood flow left. Blood supply is, of course, required to heal. Michael Jackson simply had too many surgeries on his nose, causing him to lose tissue.

Another good rule to follow is exemplified in his case. If your doctor tells you no, you should definitely not do it. Some people go doctor shopping until they find one who's willing to do a procedure for them. If a doctor who is board certified and experienced in this area tells you not to have surgery, you should really listen. And if you hear the same thing from two or three people, you should definitely take the advice. Don't keep asking until you get the answer you want, because it's unlikely that you'll be happy with the results.

## BEFORE AND AFTER

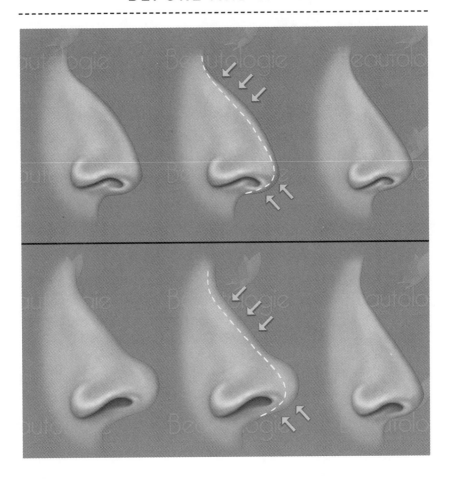

# CHAPTER 3

# Liposuction

L iposuction is the removal of fat from your body utilizing a cannula (a tube inserted under your skin) to suction the fat from unsightly problem areas that do not go away with weight loss or exercise. Liposuction is a procedure you can have performed in many different areas on the body. From the top down, you can have liposuction performed on your neck, chest, arms, abdomen through waist, hips, back, mons pubis (the area on top of your pubic bone), thighs, knees and calves.

The main reason why people opt for liposuction is because they have problem areas of fat they can't get rid of with diet and exercise. They don't like the contour of their body in that area, but no matter what they do, they just can't get rid of it. For example, many women are genetically programmed to carry some excess fat in their outer thighs, which are often referred to as "saddlebags." They may find that even at their healthy weight, they still have this area of fat that prevents their pants from fitting well. For such areas, liposuction works phenomenally well in concert with weight loss and exercise.

## The Procedure

Liposuction can be done either with a local anesthetic or a general anesthetic, under which you are totally asleep. The method of anesthesia depends on a few factors: the amount of liposuction being performed, the number and location of areas being suctioned, and the preference of the doctor performing it. Both methods, in the right hands, are safe and effective.

On the day of your surgery, your doctor will probably draw concentric circles around the areas where you want to have liposuction, before you are placed under anesthesia. Then the liposuction will be performed through tiny, linear incisions of less than half a centimeter—one for each of the areas where you're undergoing the liposuction. The incisions are so tiny that you can barely see them after a few months, in most cases. Before suctioning the fat, the doctor will first inject a fluid mixture called tumescent solution, which is a combination of saline, Epinephrine, and Lidocaine. The Epinephrine in this solution decreases bleeding during the procedure, the Lidocaine numbs the area and provides pain relief after the surgery, and the saline makes the fat more amenable to suction, making the procedure easier for the surgeon and less damaging to the body.

After an appropriate amount of tumescent solution is injected, a cannula is connected to a suction machine to suction the fat out. The physician carefully moves the cannula back and forth to contour the area that is being suctioned.

There are a couple of additional tools that can be used during liposuction today. The ultrasonic cannula uses ultrasonic waves to heat and melt the fat before it is suctioned, making it easier to withdraw, and, some say, less painful. The other tool is a laser cannula, which is used to melt the fat before removal with suction. Using these additional tools makes the withdrawal of fat less traumatic so you heal quickly and have less bruising. Your doctor will decide which of these tools should be used depending on the area being worked and his own personal preference.

## Length of Procedure

Liposuction can take anywhere from one to four hours, depending on how much fat you're having removed and from how many different areas of the body. It is very important to discuss the length of your procedure and amount that is estimated to be removed with your doctor before surgery. The American Society of Plastic Surgery recommends that no more than 5,000 cc of fat be removed in an outpatient surgery. This is very important because removal of any more fat than this without postoperative monitoring can lead to postoperative complications, a possible hospitalization, and even death.

### Noninvasive Options

Currently, a number of noninvasive options are offered to help reduce fat pockets. Fat freezing, in which we put a device on the problem area to freeze the fat underneath the skin, has gained recent popularity. In addition, radio frequency devices, which use radio frequency waves to disrupt fat cells under the skin, have also been shown to have some effect. These methodologies can be performed by nurses or a physician in an office setting. They're considered noninvasive, since no incision is made in the skin. In general, there isn't as much recovery time, but the treatments take a lot longer, and you will require multiple treatments. If you're considering this type of procedure, keep in mind that it isn't as effective as traditional liposuction. Liposuction is the direct removal of fat cells, and it is instantaneous. Noninvasive treatments are generally better suited to small areas of concern in people who are at, or close to, their ideal body weight. The effects are often variable, and many people sometimes report no effect at all. It is very important to discuss your expectations in regards to how much fat will be reduced, how many treatments you will need, and the costs, before you start a noninvasive method of fat reduction.

## Realistic Expectations

- Most important to realize is that liposuction is not a weight-loss procedure. Liposuction was designed to help reduce and contour stubborn areas of fat that are resistant to diet and exercise. After liposuction surgery, do not be surprised if you do not see many pounds come off the scale—you may only lose four or five pounds at the most. In fact, immediately after surgery, some people see their weight go up due to postoperative swelling and water retention. If you are considering liposuction to achieve a lower number on the scale, you will be disappointed. However, just because we only take off a small amount of fatty tissue doesn't mean the results can't be dramatic. Taken from the right areas, a small amount of fat removal can make you look as if we took twenty pounds off.

- Prior to your procedure, you want to get down to the best weight you can. You really want to be within ten to fifteen pounds of your ideal body weight, before surgery, to see optimal results. People who undergo liposuction while still obese are often disappointed that they do not see a significant difference.

- Patience is key. Even though you will see some immediate results with liposuction, it can take up to a year to see the final outcome because it can take that long for all the swelling and postoperative changes to resolve. In fact, because of the swelling, you will actually weigh more, not less, immediately after surgery. It can sometimes be frustrating in the first few weeks after surgery when your clothes fit you more tightly than they did before the procedure. It is important, during this time, to understand that this is normal, and time will resolve these issues. I tell people not to step on the scale for at least a month after the procedure and not to worry if their pants don't close or their jeans are tight. It's all normal.

- It's also important to know that fat can come back in the same area after liposuction. When liposuction is performed, many but not all fat cells are permanently removed from the area treated. However, the few remaining fat cells can and will get larger with weight gain. If you gain weight after the surgery, the fat your body is creating will redistribute itself to all the fat cells in your body, so it won't be as apparent as before the liposuction procedure. Other areas of your body that were not liposuctioned will also preferentially gain fat if you gain weight. For example, thighs often increase in size after an abdominal liposuction.

- After having babies or losing a significant amount of weight, many people want their abdomen liposuctioned because they don't like the way it looks. The problem, in many cases, is usually loose skin, not fat. Doing liposuction in areas where you have loose skin will actually cause the area to look worse because the overlying skin will become looser as it loses the fatty tissue support. In these cases, what people really need is skin removal surgery such as an abdominoplasty (tummy tuck).

- There is a big difference between cellulite and fat. Cellulite is caused by a combination of factors directly beneath the skin, including abnormally large fat cells interspersed with bands of tissue that pull the skin down and give it the "cottage cheese" or dimpled appearance. Liposuction acts on the deeper fat levels where the cellulite doesn't really live. Cellulite is not generally treated with liposuction, and other modalities of treatment should be sought out in conjunction with liposuction.

- Some people have what is referred to as visceral fat—that is, fat on the inside of the abdomen, underneath the muscles wrapped around your large abdominal organs. This visceral fat can cause what's commonly referred to as a beer belly. Liposuction cannot be utilized to remove visceral fat because of where it's positioned: under the muscles and around your organs. If you have a large, round abdomen due to visceral fat, the only way to get rid of that is through weight loss.

### Dr. Shah Recommends

Talk to your surgeon about reutilizing the fat removed in liposuction for augmentation into the buttocks or the face. These have recently become extremely popular procedures and are generally very safe and effective!

### How to Prepare Mentally and Physically

- Foremost, you definitely want to make sure that you have your weight under control. You don't need to be at normal weight but at least at your goal weight. If your weight changes drastically after surgery, you will have a much poorer result.

- A garment or girdle is usually recommended for postoperative wear in the area where you had liposuction, so make sure you have one or two on hand. Your doctor may recommend or provide a specific garment, or you can purchase a tight-fitting garment such as Spanx™ that holds pressure in the area to prevent swelling and help contour the area. The garment is worn for about a month, postoperatively. In the beginning, you may need someone's help getting in and out of it.

- Take some time to really look at the areas where you are going to have liposuction. Notice any cellulite that may be there, and do not expect it to go away. Compare one side of your body to the other, noticing any asymmetries. Asymmetry can be helped, but it may not be completely corrected since some of it can be due to underlying bone structure or other tissues. Make sure you have "before" pictures of yourself so you can evaluate your results more realistically afterward.

### Recovery and Results

Remember that even though the incisions used for liposuction are tiny, the entire area where the fat is being removed from under the skin is affected by the procedure, which can be fairly large. The small incisions heal fairly quickly, but you're likely to have bruising, swelling, and tenderness across the entire surgical area for quite some time. Depending on the amount of fat removed, you need to give yourself at least a week to recover to the point where you feel well enough to resume daily activities. The bruising can take about two to four weeks to resolve. Do not be alarmed if the bruising seems to "move" around or go to areas where there was no liposuction performed. This is due to gravity. Swelling takes about a year to fully resolve. However, most of it dissipates in the first month after surgery. Exercise can generally be resumed about a month after surgery, but you should follow your doctor's specific recommendations.

## Risks

- *Waviness, wrinkling, or dimpling of the skin:* As technology has improved, this potential problem has become much less common. The use of much smaller cannulas (tubes inserted to remove the fat cells) has helped tremendously. Tight and firm skin before surgery will probably remain so after healing. If your skin is loose, wrinkled, or dimpled before surgery, it may remain the same or be slightly worse after surgery since the supporting fat has been removed. Much of this depends on your own skin's elasticity and time.

- *Skin tightening:* After liposuction of any area of your body, we cannot guarantee the amount of skin tightening you will have. This depends on many factors: your genetics, your skin elasticity and condition, and how much you exercise after surgery. You might require removal of excess skin (i.e., tummy tuck or other procedure) if you still feel that you have too much loose skin.

- *Asymmetry:* It is not possible to obtain perfect total symmetry when bilateral procedures are performed. Very few people are totally symmetrical prior to liposuction. If a significant difference is visible following healing, a secondary "touch up" procedure may be indicated to minimize such a condition.

- *Loss of sensation:* Usually, any numbness or loss of sensation is temporary and resolves within a few months. You may have some permanently numb areas, but this is rare.

- *Indentation or excess fat removal:* Although this can occur in an attempt to remove as much fat as possible, careful discussion and preoperative care makes this an unlikely possibility. Sometimes, fat atrophy, caused by poor blood supply or smoking, may also lead to indentations and contour irregularities. Additional procedures such as fat reinjection may be needed to correct them if they are significant.

- *Fluid and electrolyte problems:* When we anticipate that large volumes of fat need removal (5,000 cc or more), we may require you have the surgery at the hospital, depending on your overall health and age. We may require you to get additional IV fluids to help your body adjust to the loss of fluid and blood that occurs during surgery and because of the postoperative shift of fluids to the areas under the skin that were suctioned. Severe fluid and electrolyte problems, usually associated with large-volume liposuction, can cause surgical shock, require hospitalization, and, in the most extreme case, cause death. Blood transfusions may also be required. This is extremely rare if we keep to a safe volume of liposuction.

- *Infection:* This is a very unusual and rare problem. If it occurs, antibiotics will be prescribed and cultures obtained if needed. You may need to be hospitalized, but this is rare.

- *Bleeding and bruising:* Some bruising almost always surfaces for two to three weeks after liposuction. Formation of hematomas (blood clots under the skin) is rare. Resolution occurs with time and massage. Extremely rare cases may require suction of the blood clots.

- *Skin loss:* Skin loss following liposuction is extremely rare and may require secondary reparative surgery.

9. *Lumps or firmness under the skin:* During the healing phase (several weeks or longer) you may feel firmness or lumpiness under the treated areas. This is normal and will resolve with time.

10. *Seroma formation:* Fluids can collect under the skin, following liposuction (very uncommon). If this problem occurs, aspiration with a needle or even open drainage might be indicated.

11. *Pulmonary embolism:* This is a very rare and potentially fatal complication of all large operations. Fat droplets in the blood stream are trapped in the lungs and may cause breathing difficulty. Should this unlikely complication occur, hospitalization and other treatment may be necessary.

- *Deep venous thrombosis:* This is also a rare complication, usually due to prolonged inactivity. You must get out of bed after surgery and walk around the room at least three to four times a day. If you get a blood clot, you may need blood thinners. Blood clots can lead to pulmonary embolism as well, but again, this complication is rare.
- *Alternatives:* Liposuction is entirely elective. Alternatives include weight loss and exercise. Loose skin and fat can sometimes be excised with excisional procedures such as tummy tucks and brachioplasty. Alternative surgical treatments have their own potential risks. And there is always the option of doing nothing at all.

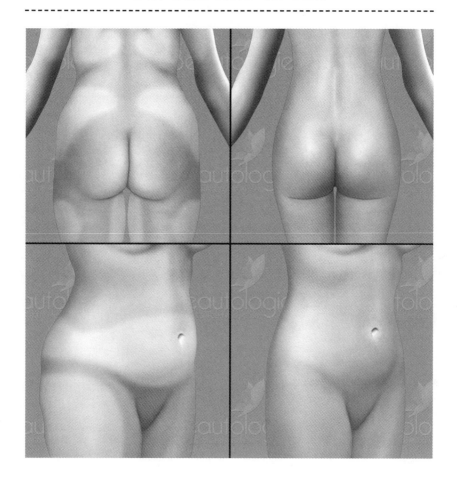

------------------------

# CHAPTER 4

# Tummy Tucks

A tummy tuck, also known as abdominoplasty surgery, is one of the most commonly sought-after procedures at a plastic surgeon's office. In its most basic form, it involves removing excess skin and stretch marks from the abdominal area, tightening the abdominal muscles, and perhaps, utilizing some liposuction to complement the results. The majority of people who seek out this procedure do it after they've given birth or after having lost a significant amount of weight, either naturally or through bariatric surgery.

## The Procedure

The incision of the typical tummy tuck goes from hip to hip. However, this can vary greatly due to your body habitus and the preference of the surgeon. Your surgeon will try to keep the incision as low on your body as he/she possibly can so it's hidden beneath the bikini or underwear line. If there is a large amount of skin to remove, the incision can extend even farther than from hip to hip to remove skin on your sides. This procedure may be referred to as an "extended" tummy tuck. Some people, typically due to bariatric weight-loss surgery, have lost so much weight and have so much excess skin that it makes sense to remove skin circumferentially from the torso. This procedure is referred to as body-lift surgery.

The next step in the abdominoplasty is the tightening of the abdominal muscles. Stretching of the abdominal wall from the inside causes your rectus muscles to spread apart from each other. This is referred to as a diastasis of the muscles and is what causes the bulging of the abdomen. We can tighten the muscles by using sutures to pull them closer to each other. Once we've done that, the next step is to carefully remove and discard all the excess skin.

A mini tummy tuck is a procedure whereby you have only a small amount of skin removed, usually about one or two inches, right above the pubic area. This usually leaves a shorter scar. Very few people are candidates for a mini tummy tuck. Typically, to have a mini tummy tuck, your BMI must be less that twenty-five, you must have no excess skin above your belly button, and you must have no muscle separation.

### Length of Procedure

A tummy tuck usually takes about two to three hours to perform under general anesthesia. A mini tummy tuck takes less time, whereas an extended tummy tuck can add another hour or more to the procedure.

### Realistic Expectations

Tummy tucks are *not* weight-loss surgeries. Generally, we only take off about two to four pounds of skin. We're not taking off so much that you're going to see a huge difference on the scale. And initially, because of the swelling, you might even weigh more than you did before surgery. You will not lose twenty pounds with a tummy tuck, and it's going to take a while before you see a reduction on the scale. After about a month of recovery and your doctor's clearance, it is extremely important that you start exercising and watching your diet. I recommend getting on the scale once a week to see how your weight is trending. Many patients tend to gain weight after these surgeries because they are stuck in "recovery mode" and convince themselves that it is somehow okay to eat as much as they want because of the surgery. Nothing could be further than the truth.

You're going to have the same abdomen after surgery, only with less skin and a tighter core. A tummy tuck doesn't make someone who is five feet five inches tall and weighs 180 pounds look like a tall and thin model. You can't give yourself the look of six-pack abs with a tummy tuck. The surgery will make your abdomen look nice and flat, but there's a big difference between that and looking as if you have 5 percent body fat. Do not expect a six-pack or a reduction in body fat with a tummy tuck.

Of course, all the stretch marks in the skin that was removed will be gone. The stretch marks above the skin removal and on your sides will still be there. It is important to know where your stretch marks are on your body so that afterward, you do not think the surgery caused them. A tummy tuck does not cause new stretch marks.

Listen to your plastic surgeon about what kind of tummy tuck is best for you. Many people insist on a mini tummy tuck because they feel it will be less invasive. A mini tummy tuck will give you mini results, and you will be very disappointed. In reality, a real tummy tuck and a mini tummy tuck are very similar in terms of the length of your incision and your recovery. If your doctor says you are not a candidate for a mini tummy tuck, do not pursue one.

The length of your incision can never be guaranteed before surgery. Your surgeon will try to make it as low and as short as possible, but during surgery, we must make the incision as long as we need to remove your loose skin.

After surgery, do not expect to be able to bend forward or sit down and not have any loose skin. You need this skin in order to stand up straight. A few patients come in after surgery and show me excess skin as they bend fully forward or assume a strange position. I tell them that there is no way we can remove so much skin that none is left to pinch, especially when they bend forward.

Your lateral flank area, or your love handles, will still be there after surgery. We can liposuction them to make them look flatter, but you will still be able to grab some skin in that area afterward. Remember that we are not excising skin there, so you will still be able to grab skin in that location.

Everyone has natural asymmetries from one side of the abdomen to the other. Often, people don't notice them before surgery, but because patients spend an inordinate amount of time in front of the mirror after plastic surgery, these asymmetries will reveal themselves. Accept them as normal; there is no reason to try to achieve perfect symmetry.

It's important that patients have realistic expectations of what can be achieved, but in reality, most patients just love their tummy-tuck results. They often say a tummy tuck is one of the best things they've ever done in their lives. Childbirth and weight loss can really damage the muscles and make women feel they're fat when they're not. A tummy tuck can help people get their confidence back and look great in a bathing suit and clothes.

## How to Prepare Mentally and Physically

Getting yourself in the right physical condition is a major prerequisite for this procedure. A lot of people think a tummy tuck is a weight-loss procedure, but it's not. A tummy tuck really just removes loose skin. You have to get your weight down to where you feel comfortable before you have one. We usually recommend that your body mass index be below thirty before a tummy tuck. Your body weight needn't be ideal, but it must be at least below thirty on the BMI scale. On a case-by-case basis, we may require even more weight loss before surgery. Afterward, you should be prepared to continue a good exercise and diet routine to maintain the results. If you have had weight-loss surgery, you want your weight to be stable for six months before you have surgery to remove any loose skin. If you're still losing weight, you shouldn't have it done. It takes about a year or more after a gastric bypass or other weight-loss procedure before most people can have plastic surgery.

You should consider whether or not you're done having children before you have a tummy tuck because getting pregnant can stretch out the skin and muscles again. If you plan to have more children, it is smart to wait until after giving birth to have the surgery.

Tummy tucks have a longer recovery period than some other surgeries, so you really want to prepare yourself for being sedentary for a period of time. People who think it's going to be a quick, easy aftermath will be disappointed. For the first two weeks, you really can't do much of anything and should just be in "vacation mode" at home. You will need help getting around, someone else will have to do all the housework, and you will need a driver.

Although this surgery results in a longer scar than other surgeries do, we take special care to hide it as well as possible. Make sure you've talked with your doctor about the location of the scar and about how to properly care for your scar. Also, prepare yourself for what it's going to look like immediately afterward by asking your doctor if you can see pictures. Patience and vigilance are the keys to being happy with any surgical scar. You need to continuously remind yourself that it's going to fade and that many patients end up with what just looks like a pencil-thin white line, after a time. Vigilance is required on your end to properly care for your scar according to your doctor's recommendations. If your surgeon has not given you advice on scar care, you should ask about it.

Abdominoplasty results also take time, mostly due to the effects of swelling. The normal postoperative swelling that occurs with this procedure goes away very slowly. Only about 30 to 40 percent of the swelling goes away in a month, and the rest takes approximately one year to go away. Prepare yourself for a year-long process. You will see the immediate results of losing stretch marks and that flap of skin, but the beautiful contouring only happens after you have given the swelling an opportunity to resolve itself.

## Recovery and Results

Women who have had a C-section will have an idea of what a tummy tuck feels like. It's hard to get up, get yourself out of bed, and stand up straight for a few days to weeks. If you've had your muscles tightened, you'll also feel full quickly and won't be able to eat as much. For a about a week, you will probably need some help to move around. You will feel faint and dizzy for a couple of days, so it is imperative that you have someone at home to help care for you.

If you have a desk job, you're going to need to take at least two weeks off work after the procedure. If any physical activity is involved in your job, you'll want to give yourself four to six weeks off.

After surgery, you will most likely have a drainage tube that comes out the side of your incision and removes excess fluid. There's a suture that holds the tube in place so it doesn't fall out. The other end of the tube is attached to a JP bulb, which is a small plastic suction container that is the size and shape of an egg. You'll need to empty it periodically, and it is generally removed after a week or two.

Exercise routines can usually be started four to six weeks after surgery. Having to stay away from the gym can be difficult for some patients because they've often worked hard to lose weight prior to their surgery. They feel as though they don't want to get out of their routine, regain weight, and diminish the slimming effect of the surgery. My advice is to go for a walk instead, as tolerated. Replace the gym routine with a different one temporarily. Giving your body the correct amount of time to heal is imperative. Going back to the gym too early can delay your healing for months if a complication develops.

### Risks

- *Incisions (scars)*: After a full abdominoplasty, you will have a long scar above the pubic hairline extending toward the flanks or beyond, as well as a scar around the umbilicus (belly button) and possibly a shorter vertical scar in the midline, just above the pubic hairline.

  - Due to the low placement of the incision, and variability in every patient's skin elasticity, the pubic hairline may become elevated. Usually this can be hidden by underwear, but occasionally permanent or temporary hair removal may be necessary. You should discuss your incision lines with your surgeon and plan the incision to accommodate, within limits, different clothing and bathing-suit styles. In cases of extreme skin redundancy, where a vertical abdominoplasty is also performed—that is, after massive weight loss—a vertical scar extending from the pubic hairline to the lower end of the breastbone may result. If you have chosen an extended abdominoplasty, the scars will extend around the hips toward the back.

- After an abdominoplasty, you always have the possibility of a vertical scar because of the inability to remove the old umbilicus location due to lack of skin. We may not be able to tell you that this is a possibility before surgery because we don't know the true elasticity, or "pull," of your skin until we are in surgery.

- If you are having a mini-abdominoplasty, we may not be moving your umbilicus, so you will not have a scar around your belly button. The horizontal scar above the pubic hairline will be shorter than the scar after a full abdominoplasty.

- Redness, thickness, and some widening of these scars to a variable extent will occur once you return to normal activities. Incisions placed in high-tension areas (i.e., abdomen, shoulders, knees) tend to create slightly wider scars. We will work with you to minimize these scars but can make no guarantees on how your scar will heal, how long it will be, how high it will be, and if it will heal properly. You may need a scar revision, laser, or other treatments if you are not satisfied with the scar. You are financially responsible for all of these treatments.

- *Uneven skin contours:* Following an abdominoplasty, the skin contours may be slightly uneven and areas of slight depression or wrinkling can occur. As healing progresses, most of these problems (if present) usually improve dramatically. If after one year there are still areas that are uneven, and we can show that you have lost weight since your surgery, additional liposuction can be done to improve these contours.

- *Asymmetry:* Some asymmetry of abdominoplasty scars and contours occurs frequently as healing is not always even from side to side. Also, it is important to realize that we are not built symmetrically to start with, and these natural asymmetries may be more noticeable after surgery. Mild asymmetry is usually not cosmetically significant. If the asymmetry is significant, revisional surgery may be considered.

- *Belly button (umbilicus):* The belly button may be slightly off center, heal poorly, suffer necrosis (loss of circulation), protrude, or be unusually retracted. Significant problems are uncommon. After one year, if you and the surgeon agree there is a problem, it may be corrected with a minor procedure.

- *Loss of sensation:* Usually, any numbness or loss of sensation is temporary and resolves within a few months. It may take up to a year or longer to get full recovery of your nerve sensation. During the recovery process, you may notice oversensitivity, burning, or electrical-shock sensations. These are all normal symptoms and will resolve over time. If sensation does not fully return, there is nothing that we can do to make it come back, and you will be permanently numb in those areas.

- *Fat necrosis:* In rare cases, some of the underlying fat can necrose (die) because of infection, excessive tension due to over activity, or poor health. An uncommon problem, it is usually nothing more than an annoyance, requiring additional healing time, dressing changes, and possible revision, later. It is unlikely to seriously affect the ultimate outcome but may result in some wide scars that require revision.

- *Skin loss:* As with fat necrosis, skin loss can result from infection or excessive tension due to overactivity. The treatment is the same regardless of the cause. Careful preoperative planning and resisting the urge to make the tummy as tight as possible reduces but does not eliminate the possibility of this problem. Dressing changes and time will be required to heal skin loss, and possibly, additional surgery.

- *Dog ears:* When your surgeon closes the angle at the end of the skin incision during the repair, a projection of bulging tissue called a dog ear can occur. Liposuction under the area or extension of the incisions can solve or reduce the problem. If a small dog ear appears at the end of surgery, it will usually flatten or disappear with time and healing. If it remains visible, a small procedure under local or general anesthesia can solve the problem at a later time. Usually, time will correct the problem on its own. If not, we generally wait six months to treat this problem. Dog ears are very common, and they are not a complication. They are simple to repair and are always removed by your surgeon when the time is right.

- *Fat emboli and blood clots:* These problems can rarely occur with any surgery, but they occur a little more frequently after an abdominoplasty. Shortened operating time, postoperative leg movements, and walking soon after surgery help to avoid these problems. Although fat emboli and blood clots can be life threatening, they usually resolve completely with hospitalization and care by a medical specialist, who will probably prescribe blood thinners for some months.

- *Fluid accumulation (seroma):* Rarely, tissue fluids collect under the abdominal skin flap (usually after the drains have been removed). If this occurs, aspiration of the fluid with a needle two or three times a week for a few weeks usually solves the problem. Few patients require further surgery or replacement of the tube.

- *Liposuction risks:* Generally, liposuction is used at the time of a tummy tuck. This can cause bruising, uneven contours, lumpiness, and swelling, which almost always resolve with time.

- *Weight gain/dissatisfaction with results:* It is important to have realistic expectations after an abdominoplasty. During your tummy-tuck procedure, your surgeon will remove as much skin and tissue as possible. An abdominoplasty will not reduce your overall body fat percentage to a degree that will make you skinny and does not take many pounds off the scale. Although you will certainly look as if you have lost many pounds, the results may only be noticed when your clothes are removed. It is essential to know that a tummy tuck must be combined with good eating habits and exercise to promote overall weight loss and BMI reduction. If you are still not satisfied with the way you look after a tummy tuck, the only solution is to lose weight and exercise as much as possible to reduce your BMI to less than twenty-five and tone your skin and muscles as much as possible.

### Dr. Shah Recommends

Starting one month after a tummy tuck, a smart idea is to weigh yourself weekly. You should see the weight slowly creep downward due to the loss of swelling. If your weight is staying or going up, it's time to start moving! Your lack of activity is causing you to gain weight again!

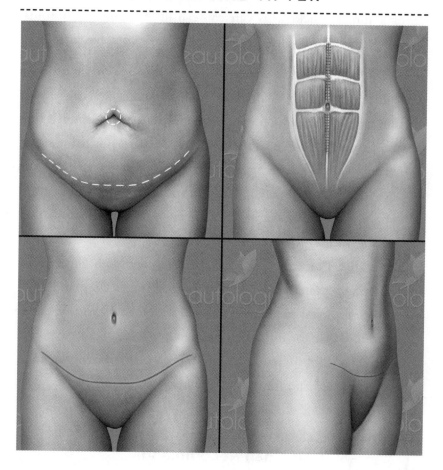

CHAPTER 5

- - - - - - - - - - - - - - - - - - - - - -

# Breast Augmentation

B reast augmentation is one of the most popular plastic surgery procedures performed today. The procedure has become more socially acceptable over the last two decades, and many women now consider the procedure to be almost "expected" after childbirth and breastfeeding. Women get breast augmentation for several different reasons, but the most popular reason is that after having a baby and breastfeeding, women tend to lose breast tissue and the breasts look somewhat "deflated." This happens because of hormonal changes that occur when women finish breastfeeding and the body signals the breast tissue to stop producing milk. Breast augmentation can refill the breast, giving it back the fullness and perkiness that was present before breastfeeding.

Another common reason to pursue breast augmentation is simply unhappiness with body shape. A woman may think her breasts are too small for her body or their shape doesn't appeal to her. Asymmetry, meaning the breasts are different sizes, may also be a factor. Some asymmetry is normal, but noticeable differences can be helped with this surgery.

Finally, there's the whole area of reconstructive breast surgery after tissue has been removed due to cancer. We can use implants as part of the reconstructive surgery to regain the breast volume lost at the time of resection.

Because of the thousands of media impressions, websites, and anecdotal stories women hear almost every day, breast augmentation tends to be the procedure giving surgeons the most problems with patients' unrealistic expectations. This means there should be a lot of communication between the doctor and patient as far as what the patient wants versus what can realistically be accomplished. It's one of those procedures in which the surgeon has the ability to modify the end result based on the desires of the patient. The surgery is also unique in that the patient has many options available, and it is the doctor's job to help the patient choose the correct options for her. Keep in mind, however, the surgeon is limited by the amount of space you have on your chest and the elasticity of the skin.

## The Procedure

A breast augmentation starts with a small incision, about an inch long, made underneath the fold of the breast, in the armpit, or around the areola. Choosing the incision site is something you will do in partnership with your doctor. After the incision is made, a pocket is made for the implant either under or above your breast muscle. The location of the implant involves another decision you will arrive at with your doctor. The most common strategy for placing an implant is to make an incision under the breast and also under the muscle.

There are two major categories of implants: saline and silicone. You have to decide what's right for you through a dialog with your doctor. Saline implants are filled with salt water. Silicone implants are filled with a cohesive silicone gel. You may have heard about the older implants filled with liquid silicone, which caused health problems, but the FDA took those silicone implants off the market. Since then, silicone implants have been completely redesigned. Now they're filled with a cohesive gel, which is much safer. Basically, you can cut the implant in half and the gel still sticks together instead of leaking as the old implants used to.

Most patients prefer to use the silicone implants because they're softer, they feel more natural, and they achieve a more natural shape. They are definitely the most popular implant type chosen. The decision regarding the kind of implant used, however, is ultimately decided by you in partnership with your surgeon. Regardless of which you choose, the surgical processes are essentially the same.

The saline implant comes empty from the manufacturer and is rolled and inserted through a small incision. After the implant is placed, it is filled with saline. The silicone implants come prefilled, but they're flexible, and the doctor folds them to fit them through the incision.

After the implants are placed, the doctor will confirm that the implant is in a good position and close the incision with sutures under the skin in multiple layers.

### Length of Procedure

A breast augmentation takes about one to two hours, but the duration can vary depending on the complexity of the procedure.

### Realistic Expectations

- Many people assume that having breast implants will result in the giant breasts that Pamela Anderson sported in *Baywatch*. In reality, that type of result is rare. In fact, most breast augmentations are not noticeable to the public. You would be genuinely surprised at how many people have had a breast augmentation done with implants that fit their body frame, resulting in a totally natural look. In some cases, patients ask for large breasts, "I don't want it to look natural. I want it to look fake. I want people to notice I have them." That's just their preference. Pamela Anderson and others like her chose to get really large implants, but they are not at all representative of what implants look like on most people. This is why it is important to communicate your desires honestly with your surgeon. If you want large, fake-looking breasts, make sure you tell your surgeon. If you want natural-looking breasts, it is important to make that known too. Also know your friend's or colleague's large breast implant surgery was likely not recommended by the surgeon. More often than not, it was the patient's choice to have large breasts. I often hear, "I didn't want to go to Dr. X because he makes them too large!" In reality, that patient may have just seen one or two of Dr. X's patients who happened to have requested the large look.

- Many women misunderstand how the skin on their breasts will look after surgery. When viewing before and after photos online, you should realize that someone who wears an A-cup bra and has practically no breast tissue and tight skin will have a stretched, tight look after placement of a breast implant. Often, the breast doesn't hang over the breast fold. It looks like a round ball under stretched skin. However, someone who starts with C-cup sized breasts and a good amount of breast tissue and skin is going to look much more natural after breast augmentation surgery. This is because the surgeon is simply filling the skin with the implant, versus stretching the skin. The result has everything to do with your starting point. The more you start with, the more natural you will look afterward.

- Yes, you can pick between different sizes of implants within limits. The size of a breast implant really depends on many factors: your body frame, your existing cup size, your desires, the quality of your skin, the amount of skin, and so on. Your body frame measurements are very important because the bigger an implant is, the wider it is. We can't put a really large implant in someone who's very petite because it will look abnormal and might not even fit. At the doctor's office, you will be given a range of sizes and asked to choose between different cc's (cubic centimeters of saline or silicone). Realize that a doctor's estimate of what a certain sized implant can do for your breasts and which cup size you might end up with is never a guarantee, as cup sizes vary by manufacturer.

- Implants could potentially last the rest of your life, but it's likely you will need to change them later if you want to change their size or look, you have some sagging as a result of childbirth and breastfeeding, your weight changes, or your breasts are large and heavy and sag from not wearing a bra. Also, implants may rupture at any time. Although it's not dangerous to your life to experience rupture, it does require replacement. The decision to replace your implants, and the frequency with which you do so, is between you and your surgeon.

- One of the most frequent regrets I hear after surgery is, "Oh my gosh, I wish I'd gone bigger." This often happens when patients are too scared to go to the size they want for fear of their breasts looking too large or being too noticeable. What I tell patients when they're choosing their implants is to first try them on. Most surgeons have sample sizes in their office that you can place in your bra to estimate the end result. Many surgeons also have software that can give you an idea of what the results could be. In general, it does take about a year to get used to the way your body looks, how clothes fit, and the size. Give the results a year to mature, and you may find that you did pick the perfect size to begin with!

- Many people with sagging breasts will try to place a large implant to fill the breast skin. This often results in very large, sagging breasts that now require corrective surgery. If you are seeing a true plastic surgeon, and he recommends a breast lift, then you should do the lift! Just placing implants could make the problem much worse!

- Your cleavage is determined by many factors. The largest determinant of how much cleavage you will have (the space between your breasts) is how far apart your breasts are to start with. This is the "footprint" of your breast, which is a combination of your overall body frame, the width of your sternum (breast bone), and the shape of your sternum. The breasts cannot be "moved" on your chest wall, so there are limits to where we can place the implant. Of course, no matter what, you will see an improvement in your cleavage.

### How to Prepare Mentally and Physically

- First and foremost, you must ensure that you have had an in-depth consultation with your doctor to communicate what you're looking for. You should be proactive and forthright in your discussion. You might want to get pictures, especially before and after pictures, that look like your body in the before photos and show the results you want to achieve in the after pictures. You can find such pictures online or on plastic surgery websites. Some people bring in magazine photos, but you should know that in magazine photos, people wear bras and clothes that change the shape of their breasts. It's better to get natural pictures from plastic surgery sites to get a real representation of what the results will look like. Have a list of questions prepared for your consultation. If you do not feel that you were adequately informed, or your doctor says that your desired results cannot be achieved, be sure to seek out other consultations, as well.

- It's important to find before pictures of someone who has the same amount of breast tissue and sagging as you do to get a realistic view of the potential results of implant surgery. The amount of ptosis (sagging of loose skin and breast tissue) can change the results dramatically. The more skin you have to start with, the more natural you're going to look after the implant is placed. The less skin you have, the more unnatural or stretched your breasts will look. The difference is that when, surgeons put breast implants in people who have a lot of skin, they're filling the skin versus stretching the skin of patients who have tight skin to start with. This is a very important concept for patients to understand.

- When looking at "before and after" comparisons on the Internet or in the doctor's office, you need to know one cardinal rule. If you really like the "after" but the "before" doesn't look much like you, then the "after" is unrealistic! The "before" should match not only the amount of breast skin and tissue you have but also your body type and areola position. There are a lot of variables that affect your outcome, and you should train your eyes to notice these things.

- When you're choosing the size of your implant, there needs to be effective and clear communication with your surgeon. You have to show the doctor what results you're looking for, the doctor has to measure your body frame to see what's realistic, and then you have to find some common ground between the results you want versus what is possible. If you are lucky, the results you are looking for will fall within the realm of possibility, which is the case for most people. You should expect your doctor to give you some feedback about what you're looking for and how natural it will look and whether it's even attainable. Most of the time, you will be allowed to try on an implant in the size you want or see a digital representation of the potential result.

- I encourage all patients to carefully look at their breasts in the mirror a lot before they undergo surgery so they can notice small differences and asymmetries in their breasts, such as where the right nipple is in relationship to the left nipple, the shape of both their breasts, the amount of skin on one breast compared to the other, where the right breast fold is compared to the left, and so on. Many women don't notice that they have asymmetry or unevenness before the surgery, but afterward, they look at their breasts a lot during the healing process and notice, for the first time, flaws that were there before. It is important to recognize these asymmetries and discuss with your surgeon, before surgery, the possibility of having them worked on.

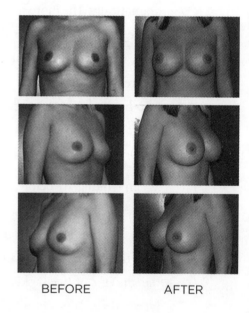

BEFORE          AFTER

- You want to prepare yourself for the fact that your breasts will look odd immediately after surgery and for a few weeks. Initially, many people are surprised that their breasts look almost square because of the swelling. They'll also look much bigger because they're high up and need to drop into place. I like to show people a picture of what they'll look like immediately after surgery so they know what to expect. This gets better, week after week and usually, after only one month, things are looking very good.

- You should really wait until you're at least eighteen years old before having implants. Your breasts do not finish developing until you're eighteen. You want your breastfeeding mechanism to fully develop so you don't interrupt that process.

### Recovery and Results

The recovery time after a breast augmentation has improved over the years as better surgical techniques have been developed. In general, most people spend a couple of days at home relaxing. During this time you will be sore, and the pain medication we give you will make you sleepy. After two to three days, most people stop taking their prescription pain medication and switch to over-the-counter pain relievers. At this time, you will find that you are able to go about your normal day, with some soreness at times. If you have a desk job, you want to take about a week off to truly ensure that you do not overdo it at work. If you have a physical job, however, your surgeon will probably want you to take at least four weeks off. During the first few weeks after a breast augmentation, you want to avoid house chores and repetitive arm movements. You should also wait at least four weeks before going to the gym.

You have to take care of the scar according to your doctor's instructions, but in most cases, only a very small incision is involved. If you take good care of it, the scar usually fades away nicely within six months to a year.

## Risks

- *Capsular contracture:* Capsular contraction (or contracture) is a possible side effect of breast implant surgery. During surgery, a pocket is created for the implant that is somewhat larger than the implant itself. During healing, a fibrous membrane, called a capsule, forms around the implant. Under ideal circumstances, the pocket maintains its original dimensions and the implant "rests" inside, remaining soft and natural. For reasons still largely unknown, however, in some women, the scar capsule may shrink and squeeze the implant, resulting in various degrees of firmness. This contraction can occur soon after surgery or many years later and can appear in one or both breasts. Capsular contraction is not a health risk, but it can detract from the quality of the result and cause discomfort, pain, or distortion of the breast contour. In cases of minor contraction, usually we will not suggest surgical correction. Cases of very firm contraction may require surgical intervention. If the contraction recurs and cannot be eliminated, which is rare, the patient may choose to have the implants permanently removed. With capsular contracture, surgeons usually try medical therapy first, to reduce the scar tissue. If that does not work, a surgical procedure (capsulectomy) may be required.

- *Hematoma:* Some postoperative bleeding into the pocket containing the breast implant occurs in 2 to 3 percent of women. If the bleeding is minimal, the body will absorb it with time. Marked swelling will probably require surgical removal of the blood. This is most often caused by overactivity and/or trauma during the recovery period.

- *Infection:* Postoperative infection is uncommon but possible. We reduce this to a minimum by giving intravenous antibiotics before your surgery. Most infections are mild and resolve without incident. If a serious infection develops, the implant will probably need to be removed and cannot be safely replaced for at least three to six months after healing.

- *Numbness:* Nerves that supply skin or nipple sensation may be cut or damaged while the space (also referred to as a "pocket") for the implant is being created. Although this does not happen routinely, it can happen no matter how carefully the surgery is performed. If sensory loss occurs, the nerves slowly recover over a period of one to two years in about 85 percent of cases. Stretching of the nerves also can cause temporary numbness.

- *Extrusion:* Thin skin, inadequate tissue coverage, capsule formation, infection, or severe wrinkling may all contribute to the erosion of an implant through the skin or scar. Should this very rare complication occur, implant removal would probably be indicated (at least temporarily).

- *Rippling:* With thin skin, placement above the muscle, or larger implants, wrinkling under the skin can be more noticeable. This is especially true with saline implants. Occasionally, the edge of the implant can be felt or seen. These problems are usually mild and require no treatment. Experience has shown that the wrinkles and ripples frequently improve or even disappear within a year. Sometimes, you may need to change to a silicone implant or a smaller implant to help treat the issue.

- *Revision:* If your breasts had slightly different shapes before surgery, they may remain slightly different after surgery. Rarely, in spite of careful attention to detail, the dissected pockets may end up slightly different in shape or height. If this is not noted while you are in surgery but becomes a problem after healing, you may need a small adjustment procedure. Sometimes, additional fluid may be added to one implant to make the size match better. Some implants may need to be repositioned after surgery to obtain better symmetry. Repositioning may be done by suturing the pocket or changing the dimensions of the pocket. This procedure is only done if the surgeon agrees that it will give you a significant improvement.

- *High implants:* Since the implants are usually placed under the muscle, they will temporarily be pulled upward. Occasionally, the implants may appear higher than their original position because of muscular contraction. This will eventually resolve, and the implants will "drop" into a better position over the next six months. Placing the implants under the muscle may reduce visible wrinkling and lead to less capsular contracture and more-natural-looking results. If the implants do not drop after a reasonable amount of time, a small revision procedure may be needed to help them achieve the correct placement.

- *Rupture:* If for any reason the valve or implant shell fails, the saline will leak and be excreted by your body. This causes no medical harm, but the implant will need to be replaced in a secondary procedure. The rate of saline implant leakage is quoted at about 1 to 2 percent over many years. If you have silicone implants, an MRI may be required to diagnose the rupture. The silicone usually stays within the implant, but it will have to be replaced. The manufacturer warranty on the implant covers the cost of the implants and may cover part of the operating fees.

- *Skin loss:* This is an extremely rare complication of breast enlargement. It usually develops from an infection that has gotten out of control and results in the death of the affected tissues. This very rare complication will usually affect only small areas that will eventually heal with good wound care. Secondary surgery is a remote possibility.

- *Breastfeeding:* Many women with breast implants have nursed their babies successfully. Nevertheless, any breast surgery can theoretically interfere with your ability to breastfeed. There is no guarantee that you will be able to breastfeed after surgery. However, submuscular placement, an incision below the breast fold, and placing a reasonably sized implant can maximize your chances of successful breastfeeding.

- *Mammograms:* In some patients, a thin layer of calcium will develop within the scar capsule surrounding the implant. This usually occurs several or more years after the implant has been inserted. In these patients, the added density of the scar may reduce the detectability of lesions close to the scar on mammograms. Breast cancers may still be visible and detectable when specialized techniques are used. There is no evidence linking implants and breast cancer. The only clinical studies available show that the prevalence of breast cancer in women with implants is the same or even slightly lower than that in women without breast implants! Furthermore, two studies have shown that the stage of breast cancer detection in women with implants appears to be identical to that found in the overall population. You should alert the technician to the fact that you have implants. Special techniques will be used and extra views may be needed in order to see as much of the breast tissue as possible. Even under the most ideal circumstances, some breast tissue may remain unseen and a suspicious lesion missed. Because the breast is compressed during mammography, it is possible, but rare, for an implant to rupture.

- *Symmastia:* This is a very unusual problem that can develop after normal augmentation either above or below the muscle. The skin over the lower sternum (breastbone) pulls away from the bone, and normal cleavage is reduced or eliminated. In its more serious form, the pockets on either side merge to form a single pocket. In the more minor form, the pockets remain separate, but the skin tents upward. Reduced fibrous or elastic "strength" in the subcutaneous tissues may be contributory but is difficult to predict. If the problem develops, correction will require secondary surgery.

- *Silicone:* Some women have claimed that silicone gel prostheses have contributed to or stimulated connective tissue disorders such as systemic lupus erythematosis, scleroderma, rheumatoid arthritis, and so on. Other complaints involving the nervous, skin, and immune systems have been reported. Reports claiming a causal relationship between silicone gel and such symptoms have been published in the medical literature and widely reported in the press. To the present time, no such relationship has been established scientifically. Saline-filled implants are made of silicone rubber. Silicone rubber has not been implicated in any diseases and has been used in many types of implants.

- *Size:* Based on your body frame, you will be recommended size choices that will fit what the surgeon feels is safe and will help you get the desired result. It is very important to know that the final cup size of your breast cannot be guaranteed in any way. If you desire a future surgery to increase the size of your implants, you may choose to add fluid to your implants or you may need to have the implants replaced with a larger size. You must wait at least six months before such a procedure. Most of the time, the surgeon will recommend that you do not go ahead with such a procedure, and if you do, you do so at your own risk. The procedure to refill an implant will weaken the implant and can cause it to wrinkle or rupture. The warranty may not be enforceable if you have this procedure.

## UNDER THE BREAST INCISION AND UNDER THE MUSCLE PLACEMENT

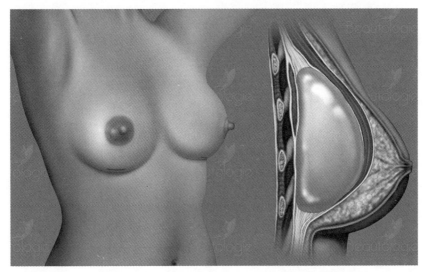

*CHAPTER 6*

– – – – – – – – – – – – – – – – – – –

# Breast Lifts and Reductions

n its most simplistic explanation, a breast lift is performed when the nipple and areola of your breast has fallen below the level of your breast fold. This occurs when there is an excess of skin on the breast, which has dropped the position of the nipple and areola to this position. The breast lift surgery is basically removing this excess skin and also lifting the nipple and areola to a new, higher location. Additional breast tissue can be removed concurrently with the lift if the patient desires. This procedure is called a breast reduction.

At the time of a breast lift, we can also use implants to fill the tissue envelope and give the breast more shape and more superior fullness. Many patients are unsure whether they need a breast augmentation or a breast lift to achieve the results they're looking for. The best way to know for sure is to be evaluated by a plastic surgeon. There are a lot of factors that go into making that decision, including the amount and quality of loose skin, the desired final shape and volume of the breast, and the size and location of the areola. The surgeon can give you a good recommendation after an office visit where measurements are made of your chest and your desires are discussed.

People come to need a breast lift after having multiple children and breastfeeding. The resultant expansion, followed by the shrinking of the breast tissue, leads to loose skin and sagging. Weight loss can also cause a similar condition since most of the breast is fatty tissue that disappears with weight loss. By contrast, people who come in for breast reduction surgery generally want the procedure because the size of their breasts causes problems for them. They often have back pain, neck pain, a grooving on their shoulders from their bra straps, and even rashes under their breasts. Or they might just not like the look of their breasts and think they're way too large because they have trouble finding bras and clothes that fit. All of these things can be helped by a breast reduction.

## The Procedures

A surgical breast lift or reduction can involve a number of different incisions depending on how much skin and tissue must be removed. Basically, the more skin and tissue there is to remove, the more incisions have to be made.

Generally, we start with an incision around the areola to move the areola upward. The nipple and areola remain attached to the tissue and blood vessels and nerves underneath. If this is all that is required, the surgery is termed a *circumareolar lift*. If more skin removal is required, another incision is usually made, going down from the areola to the fold of the breast to remove excess skin from the bottom of the breast. This is called a vertical lift or a keyhole lift because the set of incisions resembles a keyhole. If more tissue needs to be removed, an additional incision, known as the "anchor lift," is created across the bottom of your breast in the fold area. The anchor lift allows us to remove the largest amount of skin and tissue.

The type of incision you will have is the same whether you're having a breast lift or a breast reduction. The main difference between the two procedures is that the lift mostly just removes skin; a reduction removes breast tissue and fat as well as skin.

Some patients are concerned about having an incision made all the way around their areola, thinking the areola is removed from the body and then "pasted" back on. This is rarely the case. When surgeons make an incision there, the blood vessels and the nerves in the nipple and areola are maintained. So they're not taking the areola off and putting it back on. They're just moving it up while keeping it attached to the underlying blood and nerve supply.

Sometimes, a breast implant is also placed during the procedure. This is done in the middle of the surgery through the same incisions as the breast lift; no additional incisions are required.

## Length of Procedure

A breast lift or reduction can take anywhere from two to five hours in the operating room, depending on the amount of work needed and the skill and experience of the surgeon. If you were to add an implant to the surgery, additional time would be required.

## Realistic Expectations

- Quite often, patients have the misconception that getting a breast lift is going to give them the superior pole fullness (roundness at the top of the breasts) of breast implants. That's not necessarily true. The breasts will be "higher." However, the natural tissue of the breasts settles in a natural position, giving you a "natural" look. If you want the top part of your breasts to be full and round, discuss the best implants for you with your plastic surgeon.

- Some people who get breast lifts with implants think they are going to end up with the "stretched look" that occurs when breast implants are placed in patients who wear an A-cup bra and have very little breast tissue and breast skin to begin with. However, a breast lift wraps your natural skin around the implant. It doesn't stretch your skin, so the end result is more natural. This is due to extra volume of skin created by years of laxity and decreased elasticity.

- Most women have some degree of asymmetry between their breasts. If you really take some time to look at your breasts, you'll see that one nipple is usually higher than the other, one breast fold is higher than the other, and one breast is a little bigger or smaller than the other. It is important to realize that everyone has these natural asymmetries to their breasts. After surgery, you're still going to have some natural asymmetry. There's no way your surgeon can make your breasts perfectly symmetric, so don't get overly focused on making sure your breasts look exactly like each other. We have a saying in plastic surgery: "Your breasts are sisters, just not *identical twin* sisters." Some degree of asymmetry also keeps the breasts looking more natural.

- After surgery, many women spend an inordinate amount of time looking at their breasts in the mirror as they heal. This leads to focusing on concerns that were actually minor issues before surgery but that they hadn't noticed because they weren't looking that closely. I encourage women to spend some time looking at their breasts closely prior to having surgery so that they have a real picture of what they look like naturally. Discuss any issues that you notice with your surgeon, and see whether these issues can or should be addressed.

- When you undergo a breast procedure, consider that you are having two separate surgical events. You're having surgery on one side, and then on the other side. Each side will heal a little bit differently, so don't get hung up if one side hurts a little bit more or feels a little bit different for a while. It's normal for your breasts to heal and feel different during the recovery process.

- With a breast lift, it's important to understand that your surgeon is just lifting and removing the skin off the breast, not removing the breast from your body and putting it in a higher spot. So you shouldn't expect the whole mound of the breast to move higher up on your chest. Some women's breasts are attached low on their chest (look at pictures of different woman's breasts in relationship to their elbow), and after surgery, they're still going to be attached low on the chest. There's nothing that can be done to change that; this is how they were born.

- Most women's nipples and areolas are not perfectly round or symmetrical, so don't expect them to be perfectly round and symmetrical after surgery. Your surgeon will no doubt try to match the two sides as closely as possible, but again, don't expect a complete mirror image.

- A basic breast lift doesn't do anything for the actual nipple itself except to raise it. The nipple itself will remain the same size and shape. If you want that changed, you should talk to your plastic surgeon about getting an additional procedure for the nipple itself. The areola, however, is always reduced in size if it has stretched, which is very common after pregnancy.

- Some women are very concerned about how much cleavage they'll have after the surgery. If that's a concern, it's important to talk to your doctor beforehand to get a realistic picture. Some women expect their cleavage to be very deep after a breast lift, as if they're wearing a push-up bra, and that's just not realistic. Surgery cannot replicate the effects of an antigravity bra, which isn't natural anyway. After a breast lift, do not expect your breasts to look as they do with a push-up bra.

- Regarding stretch marks on the breast, some are removed with the skin that is excised during the procedure, and some get flattened out just by pulling and flattening them. Stretch marks look better with a breast lift, but not all of them can be removed.

- The timing of your surgery is critical. Many people want to get their breasts lifted and augmented immediately before spring break or summer vacation, but that's just not a good idea. You're going to have a recovery period before you can go in the ocean or a swimming pool and before you should be exposed to sun. Additionally, you've just had major surgery and what you need to do most after surgery is rest to let your body recover. Do not expect spring break or summer vacation to be a fun recovery period if you have your surgery performed on the first day of your vacation.

- It is important that you have realistic expectations about what your surgical results will look like after breast augmentation and lift (mastopexy) surgery. As part of the planning process, your doctor or nurse will show you before and after photos of previous patients as a means of demonstrating your options in selecting the size and shape of your breast implants. It is important that you look at photographs of patients with body types similar to yours; selecting photographs of patients with similar height, weight, and a similar amount of existing breast tissue will give you a better idea of what you might look like after surgery. However, it is important to understand that every person's body is individual and minute differences in anatomy that may be hard to differentiate by the untrained eye can affect the surgical results. For example, if you have more breast tissue and skin to start with, you will have a natural result. Most women who need a lift have a significant amount of breast skin and tissue and will never achieve the stretched look of someone who wears an A-cup bra and receives a large implant. No surgeon can exactly duplicate the surgical results from one patient to another.

- Asymmetry, unhappiness with breast size, poor healing, unequal nipple height, and so on may occur. For most patients, minimal differences are usually acceptable. Larger differences may require revision surgery. Your doctor will usually wait six months to one year before performing any fine-tuning type of procedure. These procedures are extremely rare in our practice, since most patients are very happy with their first surgery.

## How to Prepare Mentally and Physically

- Breast lift and reduction is considered a flap surgery, so you definitely don't want to smoke for at least a month before and a month after the procedure, as this can prevent your skin flaps from healing due to lack of oxygen.

- Be mentally prepared for where the incisions are going to be made. It's always a good idea to ask your plastic surgeon for pictures. The incisions usually fade away very nicely over time so that you can barely see or feel them, but the incisions with this surgery are typically more numerous and more apparent immediately after surgery than they are after other procedures. Don't be taken by surprise when you first look at yourself in the mirror following surgery. It's important that you have a good picture of what the procedure entails to begin with and that you remind yourself that most of the time the incisions heal extremely well if you take good care of them.

- Have a frank conversation about the magnitude of this procedure with your loved ones before your surgery. It's likely that you're going to be apprehensive after surgery, and it will help tremendously if those close to you understand how to reassure you. Your caretakers should read the appropriate chapters in this book and be realistic about how they expect your recovery to go. They can assist by saying things such as, "It's going to be okay . . . remember the incisions will fade in time . . . you just have to wait for things to settle."

- This is one of the more complicated surgeries that are performed by plastic surgeons. You must be sure your surgeon is a real plastic surgeon who has a lot of experience doing the procedure. Ask your surgeon if he is board certified and how many of these procedures he has performed.

- If you're considering a breast reduction, you need to think about the size your breasts will end up being after the procedure. This can be hard for patients to picture, so have a conversation with your doctor about it. Some women who want a reduction are so tired of their breasts being oversized that they'll say something such as, "I hate them. Just cut them off completely and make me an A cup." But in reality, if you did that, you probably wouldn't be happy in the end. So listen to your doctor's counsel, and try to think about what you would want long term and what would make you comfortable.

- You also want to think about whether or not you're done having children. There can be problems with breastfeeding after a reduction or a lift, and if you are considering more children in the future, and breastfeeding is important to you, then it may be wise to hold off.

### Recovery and Results

The procedure generally takes about two to five hours in the operating room, depending on the complexity of the procedure and the skill of the surgeon. These surgeries are usually performed on an outpatient basis, which means you are allowed to go home and recover after the procedure. For the first few days, you will be sore, and you will be taking pain medication that will make you sleepy.

It will take approximately a week before you feel you're able to resume normal activities and go back to work if you have a desk job. It will be about a month before you begin to feel totally normal again. If you have a job that involves heavy lifting, you will want to take four to six weeks off.

Taking care of your incisions is a process that you will need to adhere to for six to twelve months to achieve optimal scars.

Occasionally, after these procedures, you'll have a drainage tube from each breast, for a few days, to remove excess fluid. There's a suture that holds them in place, so they don't fall out, and they're attached to a bulb, a small, round, egg-shaped device that holds suction on the tube. You'll need to empty the bulbs periodically and measure the output. Generally, the drainage tubes stay in for a few days, after which time your doctor will remove them, which is a pretty painless process.

After surgery, you won't be able to wear a regular bra for a period of time. You'll be given a surgical bra or be told to wear a supportive sports bra.

Be prepared to stay out of the sun, and don't go to tanning booths for a few months. If you're outside, make sure your breasts are well covered.

Stay out of swimming pools, hot tubs, and the Jacuzzi for at least a month to help avoid infection. Taking a shower is usually okay after thirty-six hours.

### Risks

- *Capsular contracture:* Capsular contraction is a possible side effect of breast implant surgery. During surgery, a pocket is created for the implant that is somewhat larger than the implant itself. During healing, a fibrous membrane called a capsule forms around the device. Under ideal circumstances, the pocket maintains its original dimensions and the implant "rests" inside, remaining soft and natural. For reasons still largely unknown, however, in some women, the scar capsule may shrink and squeeze the implant, resulting in various degrees of firmness. This contraction can occur soon after surgery or many years later and can appear in one or both breasts. Capsular contraction is not a health risk, but it can detract from the quality of the result and cause discomfort, pain, or distortion of the breast contour. In cases of minor contraction, surgical correction is not usually suggested. Cases of very firm contraction may require surgical intervention. It is rare, but if the contraction recurs and cannot be eliminated, the patient may choose to have the implants permanently removed.

With capsular contracture, medical therapy is the first line of therapy to reduce the scar tissue. If that does not work, a surgical procedure (capsulectomy) may be required.

- *Hematoma:* Some postoperative bleeding into the pocket containing the breast implant occurs in 2 to 3 percent of women. If the bleeding is minimal, the body will absorb it with time. Marked swelling will probably require surgical removal of the blood. This is most often caused by overactivity and/or trauma during the recovery period.

- *Infection:* Postoperative infection is uncommon but possible. The risk is reduced to a minimum by giving intravenous antibiotics during surgery and oral antibiotics after surgery. Most infections are mild and resolve without incident. If a serious infection were to develop, the implant would probably need to be removed and could not be safely replaced for at least three to six months after healing.

- *Numbness:* Nerves that supply skin or nipple sensation may be cut or damaged while the pocket or space for the implant is being created. Although this does not happen routinely, it can happen no matter how carefully the surgery is performed. If sensory loss were to occur, the nerves would slowly recover over a period of one to two years in about 85 percent of cases. Stretching of the nerves also can cause temporary numbness.

- *Hardness within breasts:* Postoperative scarring within the breast tissue may cause areas of hardness. Occasionally, these lumps may require mammography or even biopsies to rule out any malignancy.

- *Extrusion:* Thin skin, inadequate tissue coverage, capsule formation, infection, or severe wrinkling may all contribute to the erosion of an implant through the skin or scar. Should this very rare complication occur, implant removal would probably be indicated (at least temporarily).

- *Asymmetry and size:* No patient is perfectly symmetrical from one side to the other. Although your doctor will try to achieve better symmetry for you, you may still notice some minor differences between your two breasts. This is normal and usually correction is not warranted. Most people can never achieve perfect symmetry. We will work with you extensively to select a size before surgery. This includes our measurements, recommendations, and your trying on the implants. If you are at all disappointed with the size of your breasts after surgery, you may opt to have another procedure. Of course, the final breast size cannot be guaranteed in any way.

- *Rippling:* With thin skin, placement above the muscle, or larger implants, wrinkling under the skin can be more noticeable. Occasionally, the edge of the implant can be felt or seen. These problems are usually mild and require no treatment. Experience has shown that the wrinkles and ripples frequently improve or even disappear within a year. Sometimes you may need to change to a silicone implant or a smaller implant.

- *Revision:* If your breasts had slightly different shapes before surgery, they may remain slightly different after surgery. Rarely, in spite of careful attention to detail, the dissected pockets may end up slightly different in shape or height. If this is not noted while you are in surgery but becomes a problem after healing, you may need a small adjustment procedure. If implants were placed during surgery, additional fluid may be added to one implant to make the size match better. Sometimes, an implant may need to be repositioned after surgery to obtain better symmetry. Repositioning may be done by suturing the pocket or changing the dimensions of the pocket. This procedure is only done if the surgeon agrees that it will give you a significant improvement. After some time, the effects of gravity and age may cause changes to the implant location, and this may require a new surgical procedure.

- *High implants:* Since the implants are placed under the muscle, they will temporarily be pulled upward. Occasionally, the implants may "ride" higher than their original position because of the muscular contraction. This will eventually resolve and the implants will "drop" to a better position over the next six months. Placing the implants under the muscle may reduce visible wrinkling and lead to less capsular contracture and more natural results. If the implants do not drop after a reasonable amount of time, you may need a small revision procedure to help achieve the correct placement.

- *Rupture:* If for any reason the valve or implant covering fails, the saline will leak and be excreted by your body. This causes no medical harm, but the implant will need to be replaced in a secondary procedure. The rate of saline implant leakage is quoted at about 1–2 percent over many years. If you have silicone implants, an MRI may be required to diagnose the rupture. The silicone usually stays within the implant, but it will have to be replaced. The manufacturer warranty on the implant may cover the cost of the implants and part of the operating fees above.

- *Tissue or skin loss:* During the operation, skin flaps are undermined, and the skin envelope around the breast tissue is tightened. The remote possibility exists that small or larger areas of skin or breast tissue or even the nipple can suffer from decreased circulation and can be partly or completely lost. Should this unlikely event occur, you may require extra time for healing or further surgery for closure and/or reconstruction. Smoking, diabetes, obesity, or other health issues can increase the chance of healing problems, including skin, fat and nipple loss. Be sure to have all medical problems optimized, and stop smoking before and after your surgery. This very rare complication usually involves only small areas that will eventually heal with good wound care. Secondary surgery is a remote possibility.

- *Increased risks for smokers:* Smokers have a greater chance of skin loss and poor healing because of decreased skin circulation. We will not perform this operation on smokers. You may have to submit a cotinine test one week before your surgery, and if it is positive, you may have to cancel your procedure.

- *Breastfeeding:* Many women with breast implants have nursed their babies successfully. Nevertheless, any breast surgery can theoretically interfere with your ability to breastfeed. We cannot guarantee that you will be able to breastfeed after surgery, however submuscular placement, an incision below the breast fold, and placing a reasonably sized implant can maximize your chances of breastfeeding.

- *Mammograms:* In some patients, a thin layer of calcium will develop within the scar capsule surrounding the implant. This usually occurs several or more years after the implant has been inserted. In these patients, the added density of the scar may reduce the detectability of lesions close to the scar on mammograms. Breast cancers may still be visible and detectable when specialized techniques are used. There is no evidence linking implants and breast cancer. The only clinical studies available show that the prevalence of breast cancer in women with implants is the same or even slightly lower than that in women without breast implants! Furthermore, two studies have shown that the stage of breast cancer detection in women with implants appears to be identical to that found in the overall population. You should notify the technician to the fact that you have implants. Special techniques will be used and extra views may be needed in order to see as much of the breast tissue as possible. Even under the most ideal circumstances, some breast tissue may remain unseen and a suspicious lesion missed. Because the breast is compressed during mammography, it is possible, but rare, for an implant to rupture.

- *Symmastia:* This is a very unusual problem that can develop after normal augmentation either above or below the muscle. The risk is increased by choosing a large implant, especially if you have very tight skin. The skin over the lower sternum (breastbone) pulls away from the bone, and normal cleavage is reduced or eliminated. In its more serious form, the pockets on either side merge to form a single pocket. In the more minor form, the pockets remain separate, but the skin tents upward. Reduced fibrous or elastic "strength" in the subcutaneous tissues may be contributory but is difficult to predict. If the problem develops, correction may require secondary surgery.

- *Silicone:* Some women have claimed that silicone gel prostheses have contributed to or stimulated connective tissue disorders such as systemic lupus erythematosis, scleroderma, rheumatoid arthritis, and so on. Other complaints involving the nervous system, skin and immune systems have been reported. Reports claiming a causal relationship between silicone gel and such symptoms have been published in the medical literature and widely reported in the press. To the present time, no such relationship has been established scientifically. Saline-filled implants are made of silicone rubber. Silicone rubber has not been implicated in any diseases, and has been used in many types of implants.

- *Size:* Based on your body frame, we will recommend size choices that will fit what the surgeon feels is safe and will help you get the desired result. It is very important to know that the final cup size of your breast cannot be guaranteed in any way. If you desire a future surgery to increase the size of your implants, you may choose to add fluid to your implants or you may need to have the implants replaced with a larger size. You must wait at least six months before such a procedure. Most of the time, the surgeon will recommend that you do not proceed with such a procedure, and if you do, you do so at your own risk. The procedure to refill an implant will weaken the implant and can cause it to wrinkle or rupture. The warranty may not be enforceable if you do this procedure.

- *Incisions (scars):* Using the standard technique for this procedure, you will have scars around the areola and in a vertical line from the areola to the crease below the breast, and perhaps a scar under the fold of your breast. The scars usually flatten and fade with time, but thicker and heavier scars can persist and require subsequent treatment, including surgery. Redness of the scars may continue to fade for up to two years. Your surgeon will work with you to minimize the scars over time.

- *Postoperative Sagging:* The breast skin and tissue will continue to sag with time since we cannot stop the effects of gravity on your skin. No "lift" is forever, but wearing a bra as much as possible can slow the process. You may notice that your implants are "lower" after some time, and this is a normal effect of the combination of the weight of the implants, gravity, and your skin elasticity.

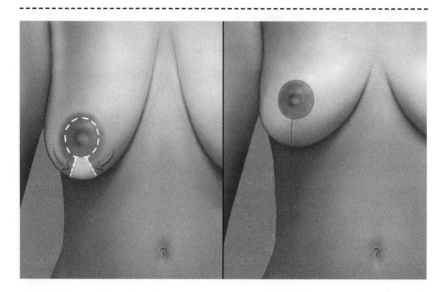

Breast Lift

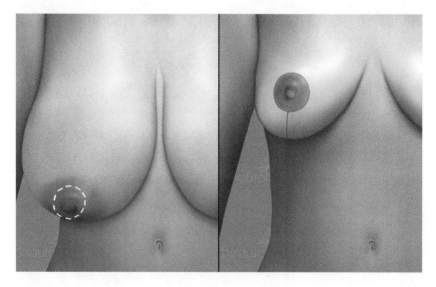

Breast Reduction

-------------------

# CHAPTER 7

# Lasers and Injectables

There are now many nonsurgical treatment alternatives that we can perform to slow down the obvious signs of aging. In fact, modern times and technology have truly changed how surgeons deal with the aging face. For many decades, the only option was a face lift, a major procedure that requires months of recovery time. Many new noninvasive procedures are now available that can be performed with almost no recovery time and at a fraction of the cost.

There are four aspects of the aging face that we can look at improving with nonsurgical tools:

1. *Fine lines and wrinkles:* Those are the little lines around your eyes or on your forehead, usually resulting from facial expression. We also call these active wrinkles since they occur with active motion of the muscles of facial expression.

2. *Deep facial lines:* These are the deeper creases that go from the nose to the mouth (nasolabial fold) as well as other

places on the face. Over time, the fine lines can become deep lines.

3. *Sagging skin and bone atrophy:* Over time, we see the effects of gravity on our face. Our cheeks, forehead, and jowls descend lower on our face as we age. This leaves hollows under the eyes, and creates jowling over time. Deeper in the face, our bone structure also tends to dissipate and atrophy.

4. *Skin quality:* With sun exposure, hormonal changes, and time, we develop age spots, red and brown spots, discoloration, unevenness, and acne scarring. All of this contributes to the overall aging of our face.

Noninvasive aesthetics can address all four of these aspects of facial aging with quick, and generally affordable procedures. The toolbox that we have in noninvasive medical aesthetics has really grown over the last ten years. It's not just Botox™ anymore! Doctors can use individual treatments or multiple treatments together to improve your overall look. Of course, treatments can still be aggressive, so you need to plan for downtime. It is also important to realize that most of these modalities are not permanent and will have to be repeated and maintained on a regular schedule.

Now let's look at the different treatment options available for each of the major categories of facial problems described previously.

## Fine Lines and Wrinkles

Currently, the best treatment for fine lines and wrinkles is a group of medications called wrinkle relaxers (a.k.a. neuromodulators) that, in very tiny dosages that are injected into exactly the right spot, prevent your facial muscles from contracting as vigorously. Preventing facial muscles from contracting keeps the skin from scrunching together, which, in turn, prevents those wrinkles from forming.

Currently, there are three different wrinkle relaxers approved by the FDA: Botox™, Xeomin, and Dysport. They are all very similar, although some doctors feel they do have slightly different indications. You should talk to your doctor and then go with whichever one he/she prefers because the differences are so subtle that you really want to empower your doctor to use whichever one he/she feels most comfortable with. All of these medications are derived from botulinum toxin. Yes, that's the same poison that causes botulism. However, remember that every medication out there is basically a poison when taken in large dosages. Botolunim toxin, injected in minute dosages into a muscle, relaxes that muscle for a period of approximately twelve weeks.

Another potential solution for fine lines and wrinkles is laser resurfacing. The treatment uses a laser to remove the top layer of skin and reveal younger-looking skin underneath. It's often reserved for people who have deeply ingrained fine lines and wrinkles that aren't completely resolved with a wrinkle relaxer. Of course, resurfacing doesn't prevent wrinkles from reforming, because your muscles are still working. It's a great treatment to do in conjunction with a wrinkle relaxer, especially if you have deeply engrained lines from years of muscle contraction.

### RECOVERY AND RESULTS

Wrinkle relaxers such as Botox are considered "lunchtime procedures." You can walk out of the doctor's office and resume your normal daily activities, and the treatment takes thirty minutes or less. It will take approximately seven days to see the full effect, and the of a wrinkle relaxer injection usually last about three to four months.

The downtime after a laser resurfacing procedure is longer, depending on the depth of the laser peel performed. However, the results are more dramatic. You can have different depths and intensities with laser resurfacing, so recovery and results really depend on which procedure you have done. After a deep laser resurfacing, your face will be very red, like a sunburn, for a couple of weeks. With some of the more superficial treatments, you may just have a few days of redness. The results of a laser resurfacing can last a year or more, depending on your skin type. It may take multiple laser procedures to get the desired result.

## Deep Lines

In addition to fine lines, your face can also develop deep lines over time. A perfect example of a deep line is the one that occurs in the nasolabial fold (a.k.a. the parentheses around your mouth), which is the fold that goes from the outside of your nostril to the corner of your mouth. For deeper lines such as the nasolabial fold, there is a whole class of injectables, referred to as fillers. Fillers come in all different sizes of molecule and are marketed under many brand names. Some fillers to consider are Restylane®, Juvederm®, Radiesse®, Sculptra®, and Aretfill®. The specific nuances of each can be explained to you by your physician.

Fillers are injected into the deep folds to fill the dermis under the fold so the fold is less apparent. These fillers can also be used in deep areas, such as your upper cheek or your lips. Amazing things are now being done with filler technology and techniques, and your doctor will be sure to offer you a myriad of options to help with a multitude of conditions that produce the appearance of aging.

Minimal downtime is needed after having an injection of any kind of filler. The injections take about fifteen minutes to an hour, depending on how many different areas are being treated and how many vials you use in one sitting. Keep in mind that multiple vials of filler may be needed if you have a deep line or you need a lot of volume replacement. Fillers are also injected into lips to help thin lips and the fine wrinkles above and below the lips, such as smokers' lines.

Although there is some bruising and swelling with fillers, in general, the recovery is fairly easy. You can return to your normal activity or work within hours after the injection, but you may have some bruising and swelling to explain for a few days.

Most fillers last somewhere between four to six months. Some even last a bit longer. This is an important item to discuss with your doctor.

## Sagging Skin

Skin "ptosis" (the medical term for sagging) occurs for a variety of reasons. The key factor is gravity, over which we have little control. Over time, every person's face will experience some ptosis, which is mainly visualized as sagging of the malar fat pad (the fat under your eye area that falls and deepens the nasolabial fold) and sagging of the jowls. Sagging occurs in conjunction with volume loss where there is also loss of some of the fat and bone under the skin, resulting in hollowing.

To address these issues, there are certain fillers that can be injected deeper in your face to make up for the volume loss. Filling in the cheek area creates additional volume that will lift the sagging skin into a higher position.

There are also other devices that can help with volume loss. Many radiofrequency and ultrasonic modalities are used to treat the collagen underneath the skin and cause it to tighten. Radio frequency devices go by the names of Venus Freeze, Thermage®, and Aluma. Ultherapy® is the name of one ultrasonic device.

## RECOVERY AND RESULTS

Minimal downtime is needed after filler treatment, and most fillers last quite a few months, and some even longer. Some fillers do last longer and appear to build up some of your natural collagen underneath, as well. Sometimes, you'll need multiple syringes of fillers to get the effect you want, injected at intervals. Fillers can sometimes cause bruising and swelling that can take a week or so to dissipate. An appointment to have a filler procedure generally lasts between thirty minutes and an hour, and numbing cream is sometimes used to make the procedure more comfortable. The perioral area is a very commonly treated area to turn back the signs of aging and can work wonders for your overall appearance.

With radio frequency and ultrasound treatments, the results vary from person to person and are hard to quantify. You will need multiple treatments to get results, anywhere from five to fifteen, depending on how much sagging you have. These modalities are noninvasive and involve a nurse or doctor using a hand piece to create heat under the skin of your face. You will be at the doctor's office for thirty minutes to an hour, and you should be able to return to your normal duties immediately after the treatment.

It is important to remember that it is impossible to achieve the effects of a facelift surgery with these modalities if you have severe skin ptosis and volume loss. These modalities are more suitable for the individual who is early in the aging process (forties or fifties) or for the older person who does not want to undergo an invasive facelift procedure.

## Skin Quality

The quality of your skin declines and changes over time, which is the precise reason why doctors talk about skin care so much. People may develop thinning of the skin, dryness, age spots, rosacea (redness), brown spots (melasma), or even severe sun damage that could be precancerous. All these conditions have different treatment options that can be used to lessen the effects of skin deterioration on our appearance. The armamentarium includes lasers, chemical peels, and skin-care regimens.

There are literally hundreds of different options of skin-care regimens and chemical peels made for specific skin problems and skin types. There are also all kinds of lasers. An effective regimen can be constructed based on your tolerance and your budget. As with any cosmetic procedure, the quicker and larger the effect, the more recovery and cost, so you will have to decide on the best option for you.

All these modalities work on more than just the face. If you have age spots on your hands, for example, or want to improve the skin quality on your chest and cleavage, your doctor can help you with these same lasers and peels.

Cosmetic lasers can also be used to remove or improve the appearance of tattoos, unwanted hair, acne, acne scarring, other types of scars (including C-section scars), and stretch marks. There are so many options now—and more developments every year—that it is important to see a specialist who stays up-to-date on the technology to ensure you are truly being offered the best out there.

Recovery and results vary, of course, depending on which treatment or combination of treatments you choose, so you're going to have to talk to you doctor about what to expect. For example, the laser that works really well for red spots is the IPL laser (intense pulsed light) laser, and you can usually go right back to work after a treatment. But if you have a more aggressive laser procedure done, such as a CO2 ablative laser treatment, you're going to need at least a week of recovery time afterward. Of course, the deeper the treatment, the more dramatic the effect and the longer the recovery.

---

### Stretch Marks

Stretch marks are permanent tears in the collagen layers of your skin, usually due to weight gain, aggressive exercise, or pregnancy. At this time, there is no "cure" for stretch marks. I have never known any of the creams and lotions sold online and in infomercials to work. So save your money.

While there's no absolute cure, there are lasers that can help. There are lasers that can remove some of the color from stretch marks and others that actually remove the top layer of skin to help blend the skin tones. There are also surgical procedures, such as a tummy tuck, which can remove some of the skin where stretch marks appear.

---

### Realistic Expectations

- You must have a clear understanding of your budget and time commitment. Many of these treatments have little or no downtime as compared to surgery, but they also mean returning to your doctor for recurring treatments on a regular or semiregular basis. More than surgery does, these types of treatment mean establishing a long-term relationship with your doctor. You may be visiting your doctor at least every three months for maintenance, possibly even more often. It's never a one-time treatment.

- The results of noninvasive medical aesthetics are not going to be as dramatic as surgery. However, they tend to fit into people's lifestyle better. You can have dramatic results, but they will take multiple treatments, and you will need maintenance. It's like preventative medicine for your face. You will have to go in every few months and keep working on it, not just to make things better but also to maintain the efficacy of it. Again, this really is a long-term relationship.

- Everyone's skin, muscles, and tissue are different. Just because your friend had a certain result with Botox®, for example, and it lasted a certain amount of time, doesn't mean the same will be true for you. Because people are so different, things are going to work differently on different people. It really takes a good relationship with your doctor to find out what works best for you. Once you find that out, you should continue along that path.

- Many of these procedures are offered in what are commonly called medispas, or "medical spas," which are popping up all over the country. You must be really careful about who's running the medical spa. Medispas should be run by a physician, with a physician guiding your treatment plan. If it is not run by a doctor and you don't ever see a doctor, you should be very suspicious of the place. Injections and other noninvasive treatments can be given by trained nurses, but a doctor who specializes in cosmetic procedures should be supervising the treatments.

- Another reason to be careful about who is doing your cosmetic procedure is that there can be side effects if the procedure is done incorrectly. You shouldn't be lulled into a false sense of security just because these procedures are noninvasive. There have been reports of blindness occurring with some of these procedures, as well as bad burns and scars. They can be dangerous if you don't have someone who knows how to perform them safely.

- Sometimes, these treatments just aren't going to help the problem. For example, fillers and radio frequency treatments probably aren't going to help a high degree of sagging on the face. In that case, a face lift would probably be needed. That's another reason why it's a good idea to go to a place that has a good relationship with a plastic surgeon so that the provider can consider all the possible options, not just the noninvasive ones, when coming up with your treatment plan.

## How to Prepare Physically

- One of the major factors in success with noninvasive medical aesthetics is that you should stop smoking. Anything that you do in this category of noninvasive medical aesthetics is completely negated by smoking. If you're smoking, you should expect to see less-than-perfect results, and you should expect more complications.

- Along the same lines, you must be prepared to stay out of the sun before and after you have almost any of these procedures. If you're planning a Caribbean vacation where you're going to be in the sun for weeks, you really shouldn't be having a laser treatment immediately before. These procedures make your skin very sensitive and can lead to burning and scarring if exposed to the sun.

## BEFORE AND AFTER

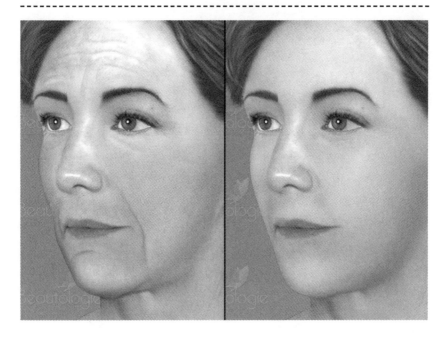

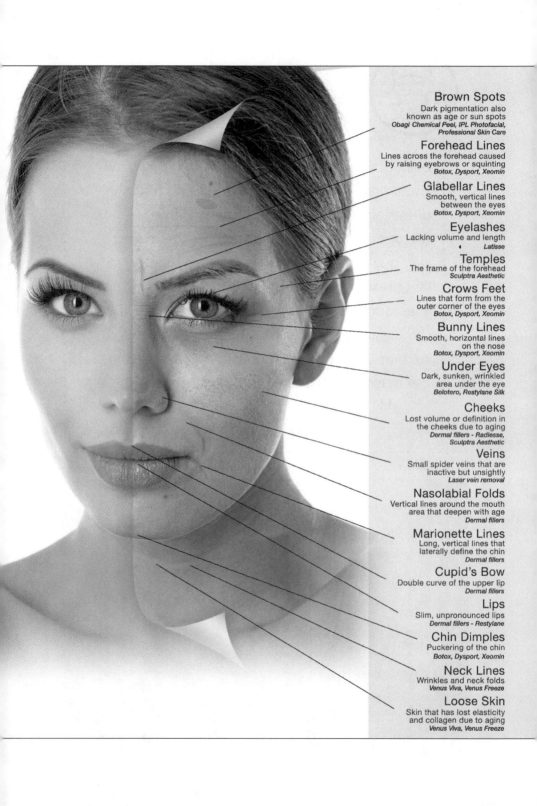

**Brown Spots**
Dark pigmentation also
known as age or sun spots
*Obagi Chemical Peel, IPL Photofacial,
Professional Skin Care*

**Forehead Lines**
Lines across the forehead caused
by raising eyebrows or squinting
*Botox, Dysport, Xeomin*

**Glabellar Lines**
Smooth, vertical lines
between the eyes
*Botox, Dysport, Xeomin*

**Eyelashes**
Lacking volume and length
*Latisse*

**Temples**
The frame of the forehead
*Sculptra Aesthetic*

**Crows Feet**
Lines that form from the
outer corner of the eyes
*Botox, Dysport, Xeomin*

**Bunny Lines**
Smooth, horizontal lines
on the nose
*Botox, Dysport, Xeomin*

**Under Eyes**
Dark, sunken, wrinkled
area under the eye
*Belotero, Restylane Silk*

**Cheeks**
Lost volume or definition in
the cheeks due to aging
*Dermal fillers - Radiesse,
Sculptra Aesthetic*

**Veins**
Small spider veins that are
inactive but unsightly
*Laser vein removal*

**Nasolabial Folds**
Vertical lines around the mouth
area that deepen with age
*Dermal fillers*

**Marionette Lines**
Long, vertical lines that
laterally define the chin
*Dermal fillers*

**Cupid's Bow**
Double curve of the upper lip
*Dermal fillers*

**Lips**
Slim, unpronounced lips
*Dermal fillers - Restylane*

**Chin Dimples**
Puckering of the chin
*Botox, Dysport, Xeomin*

**Neck Lines**
Wrinkles and neck folds
*Venus Viva, Venus Freeze*

**Loose Skin**
Skin that has lost elasticity
and collagen due to aging
*Venus Viva, Venus Freeze*

------------------------------------

# CHAPTER 8

# Hair Restoration

Some men have a genetic predisposition to balding, which can occur at any age. This problem is called male pattern baldness, and it generally begins when the hairline recedes and a patch of hairless skin starts to form on the top of the head. Eventually, those two areas coalesce and cause total baldness of the scalp.

Women are also increasingly looking into hair transplant surgery for thinning hair and eyebrows, and they can be great candidates for this procedure.

Hair transplant surgery has a bad reputation because of the old method of hair plugs. Doctors would take ten or more hair follicles at a time and move them to the front, which would look like multiple holes filled with hair plugs. The procedure has evolved tremendously since the 1980s and is now being done by replanting the hairline with one or two follicles at a time. The result is realistic and well tolerated. It is usually done under local anesthesia. Because there's artistry involved, you want to make sure you have a doctor who has a lot of experience and success in this procedure. The doctor will make decisions about where to place the hairs, even the direction the hairs go, to give you the most natural-looking appearance.

## The Procedure

The hair on a man's head that is the most resistant to balding is the hair on the back of the head. The hair transplant surgeon takes the hair from the back of the head and moves it to the front of the head by transplanting the hairs, one or two follicles at a time.

Today there are two methods for harvesting the hair from the back of the head. One technique is the strip method, which refers to a horizontal strip of hair cut out from the back of the head. Then, under a microscope, each follicle of hair is removed, one at a time, and inserted into the front of the head. This usually leaves a horizontal scar in the back of the head that is covered by the remaining hair in that location.

The second method is follicular unit extraction. During this procedure, the hair is removed from the back of the head, one follicle at a time, and moved to the front of the head. This is, of course, more time consuming, but it doesn't leave the horizontal scar of the strip method. On the other hand, the strip method takes a lot less time, and you can move a lot more hair. It's also more economical.

Hair transplants are generally done under a local anesthetic, but patients may receive sedative or intravenous medication to relax them. Patients usually watch a movie on DVD, or they'll just take a long nap. Patients also often take a break in the middle to stretch and have something to eat. The procedure can take five to eight hours, depending on the number of hairs that are being transplanted.

## Topical Treatments versus Hair Transplants

Topical treatments such as Rogaine and Propecia can work, and they're usually the first things tried by men and women who are losing their hair. The problem many people have with these treatments is that they take a long time to take effect and then they only work for as long as you use them. If you want to continue to see the effects, you'll have to keep using them for the rest of your life or your hair will go back to the way it was before you started. For those reasons, many patients choose to have a hair transplant instead.

## Realistic Expectations

- When you have a hair transplant performed, don't expect to have a full head of hair the day after the transplant. All the transplanted hairs fall out initially, and then it takes a few months for the follicles to grow new hairs.

- Because it's a long procedure, only a certain amount of hair can be moved at one sitting. How much hair is moved also depends on how much hair you have in the first place. You have to take both things into consideration when you're picturing how much hair the procedure will give you. You shouldn't necessarily expect a thick head of hair when you are done, and you may require multiple procedures over time.

- You can only do a hair transplant with follicles from another part of your head, not from any other part of your body. So people who are completely bald don't have the option of a hair transplant.

The earlier you catch and start treating your baldness, the better, so make sure to have someone check the top of your head for thinning of the hair. (You often cannot see this area in the mirror.)

## Recovery and Results

Since the procedure is done under a local anesthetic, and is not very painful, the recovery is usually only a week or less. You will be wearing a hat for a couple of weeks after the procedure, and you need to be careful about washing your head.

As mentioned previously, it will take many months for you to see the new hairs growing and filling the bald areas, so patience is key with this procedure.

## Risks

- The typical surgical risks of infection, bruising, bleeding, and swelling apply to hair transplant as they do to all surgical procedures.

- Your grafts rarely may not "take" in which case you may have to repeat the procedure.

### Men and Plastic Surgery

Most hair transplants are obviously done on men, but these days, men are also having more and more cosmetic procedures than ever before.

- In 2015 men had more than 1.2 million cosmetic procedures in the USA, accounting for 5 percent of the total.

- The number of cosmetic procedures performed on men has increased over 325 percent from 1997.

- The top five surgical procedures for men in 2015 were: liposuction, eyelid surgery, nose surgery, male breast reduction, and face lift surgery.

## NORWOOD HAIR LOSS CLASSIFICATION

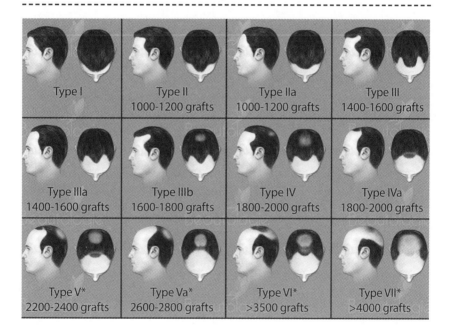

| Type I | Type II<br>1000-1200 grafts | Type IIa<br>1000-1200 grafts | Type III<br>1400-1600 grafts |
| Type IIIa<br>1400-1600 grafts | Type IIIb<br>1600-1800 grafts | Type IV<br>1800-2000 grafts | Type IVa<br>1800-2000 grafts |
| Type V*<br>2200-2400 grafts | Type Va*<br>2600-2800 grafts | Type VI*<br>>3500 grafts | Type VII*<br>>4000 grafts |

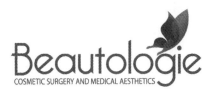

**www.beautologie.com**

### BEAUTOLOGIE—BAKERSFIELD

4850 Commerce Drive
Bakersfield, CA 93309
844-Beautologie

### BEAUTOLOGIE—FRESNO

9491 Ft. Washington Rd., Suite 101
Fresno, CA 93730
844-Beautologie

### BEAUTOLOGIE—BAKERSFIELD SOUTHWEST MEDSPA

11420 Ming Avenue, Suite 560
Bakersfield, CA 93311
844-Beautologie

### BEAUTOLOGIE—STOCKTON

4643 Quail Lakes Dr., #103
Stockton, CA 95207
844-Beautologie

### BEAUTOLOGIE—MALIBU

24955 Pacific Coast Highway c203
Malibu, CA 90265
844-Beautologie